Clinical Pathology for Athletic Trainers

Recognizing Systemic Disease

Clinical Pathology for Athletic Trainers

Recognizing Systemic Disease

Daniel P. O'Connor, MS, PT, ATC
Joe W. King Orthopedic Institute
Houston, Texas

SLACK
INCORPORATED

An innovative information, education, and management company
6900 Grove Road • Thorofare, NJ 08086

The procedures and practices described in this book should be implemented in a manner consistent with the professional standards set for the circumstances that apply in each specific situation. Every effort has been made to confirm the accuracy of the information presented and to correctly relate generally accepted practices. The author, editor, and publisher cannot accept responsibility for errors or exclusions or for the outcome of the application of the material presented herein. There is no expressed or implied warranty of this book or information imparted by it.

The work SLACK publishes is peer reviewed. Prior to publication, recognized leaders in the field, educators, and clinicians provide important feedback on the concepts and content that we publish. We welcome feedback on this work.

Printed in the United States of America.

O'Connor, Daniel P.
    Clinical pathology for athletic trainers / Daniel P. O'Connor.
        p. ; cm.
    Includes bibliographical references and index.
    ISBN 1-55642-469-8
    1. Internal medicine--Handbooks, manuals, etc. 2. Athletic trainers--Handbooks,
manuals, etc. 3. Sports medicine--Handbooks, manuals, etc. I. Title.
    [DNLM: 1. Signs and Symptoms. 2. Clinical Medicine. 3. Decision Making. 4. Disease
Attributes. 5. Sports Medicine. WB 143 O18c 2001]
    RC55 .O36 2001
    616'.0024'796--dc21

Published by: SLACK Incorporated
                  6900 Grove Road
                  Thorofare, NJ 08086 USA
                  Telephone: 856-848-1000
                  Fax: 856-853-5991
                  www.slackbooks.com

Contact SLACK Incorporated for more information about other books in this field or about the availability of our books from distributors outside the United States.

Last digit is print number: 10   9   8   7   6   5   4   3   2

DEDICATION

To Mitzi Laughlin, MS, ATC

CONTENTS

INSTRUCTORS: *Clinical Pathology for Athletic Trainers Instructor's Manual* is also available from SLACK Incorporated. Don't miss this important companion to this textbook. To order the *Instructor's Manual*, please contact SLACK Incorporated at 856-848-1000. Or visit us on the web at *www.slackbooks.com.*

ACKNOWLEDGMENTS

To Mitzi: thank you for having more patience than I deserve. I owe you (at least) 50 weekends without my "projects."

To my parents, Dan and Mary: thank you for who I am and what I have.

Special thanks to A. Louise Fincher, EdD, ATC, LAT for providing me many opportunities and for being a role model. A million thanks to Pat Lincoln and James Han, ATC for a million "little things." Thanks to Rodney Baker at the Joe W. King Orthopedic Institute for doing the thankless tasks and for his kindred sense of humor.

A very special thanks to Michael E. Cooley, BA, AMI of the Joe W. King Orthopedic Institute and Heart and Soul Illustrations for providing the beautiful illustrations.

I would also like to acknowledge several of my personal and professional mentors, all of whom I consider exceptional educators, leaders, and friends: William T. Wissen, MA, ATC, for giving me direction and discipline; Dale W. Spence, EdD, a scholar; and Allen W. Eggert, MS, ATC, for his wisdom, common sense, and patience.

Many others deserve mention for their contribution to this project. Marjorie Albohm, MS, ATC passed my original idea to SLACK Incorporated. Amy Drummond and Kate Buczko of SLACK Incorporated provided invaluable assistance from the early stages through completion. Lee Wilson and Pamela K. Henry, PT, OCS, colleagues and friends, gave me more encouragement and inspiration than they know.

I would also like to express my appreciation to the "family" of athletic trainers in the Greater Houston Athletic Trainers' Society and the Southwest Athletic Trainers' Association (NATA District 6). I am honored to be counted among your membership.

ABOUT THE AUTHOR

Daniel P. O'Connor, MS, PT, ATC, a certified athletic trainer and licensed physical therapist, received his bachelor's degree in human performance and health sciences from Rice University and his master's degree in physical therapy from Texas Woman's University. After working for a short time at the Joe W. King Orthopedic Institute, Dan became supervisor of rehabilitation at Texas Orthopedic Hospital, a position he held for 4 years. Upon enrolling at the University of Houston to pursue a doctorate in kinesiology, he returned to the Joe W. King Orthopedic Institute, where he now serves as president. He has also volunteered as a provider of onsite sports medicine coverage at events such as the Houston Marathon and the Houston Livestock Show and Rodeo.

Dan has authored several published research articles, has been invited to speak on a variety of rehabilitation and sports medicine topics at continuing education conferences, and serves as adjunct faculty at Texas Woman's University and Rice University. He has held several elected and appointed positions in the Greater Houston Athletic Trainers' Society, Southwest Athletic Trainers' Association, Texas Physical Therapy Association—Southeastern District, and is a member of the National Athletic Trainers' Association and American Physical Therapy Association. Dan also regularly participates as a test assistant for the Texas Advisory Board of Athletic Trainers (State Board of Health) and the NATA Board of Certification.

PREFACE

Clinical Pathology for Athletic Trainers: Recognizing Systemic Disease enables the athletic trainer or athletic training student to recognize and differentiate signs and symptoms produced by systemic disease. This reference book addresses the 1999 *NATA Athletic Training Educational Competencies for the Health Care of the Physically Active* related to pathology and general systemic illnesses. The NATA competencies were written with the intent of increasing the knowledge, awareness, and clinical skills necessary to identify potential systemic pathology among physically active persons.

This book provides the avenue with which to accomplish these goals. *Clinical Pathology for Athletic Trainers: Recognizing Systemic Disease* was written specifically for athletic trainers, acknowledging their unique role in the practice of sports medicine and the care of physically active people. The text will not, of course, replace a physician's examination and diagnosis, but rather presents the athletic trainer with the information necessary to make sound clinical decisions. The recognition of potential systemic illness or disease, many of which are encountered only rarely but may carry dire consequences, allows more timely and appropriate medical referral.

Clinical Pathology for Athletic Trainers: Recognizing Systemic Disease contains 12 chapters. Chapter One briefly reviews principles of clinical pathology and decision-making, such as the role of the athletic trainer, components of the medical history, and an overview of physical examination. Chapter Two, Pathophysiology, includes a discussion of homeostasis, the great biochemical stabilizing drive of the organ systems, and the mechanisms involved in inflammation and cellular response to injury. Chapters Three through Eleven outline the major diseases of the body systems, including cardiovascular, pulmonary, gastrointestinal and hepatic-biliary, renal and urogenital, endocrine, neurological, psychological, immunological, and oncological. These chapters provide a basic overview of anatomy, physiology, and pathogenesis, then discuss specific signs and symptoms, relevant medical history and physical examination findings, and clinical descriptions related to many disease states. In addition, diseases that affect sports participation, physical conditioning, and rehabilitation are also reviewed. Chapter Twelve contains evaluation and management algorithms organized by several major symptoms, thus presenting the information in the previous chapters in a clinical practice perspective. In addition, several laboratory activities outline basic physical examination techniques utilized to assess nonmusculoskeletal injuries and illnesses properly. A phonetic glossary and extensive index conclude the book.

Although primarily a practical, instructional, classroom text, many practicing athletic trainers will find *Clinical Pathology for Athletic Trainers: Recognizing Systemic Disease* to be a convenient and relatively concise reference for this very important domain of athletic training. It emphasizes clinical recognition and management of nonorthopedic pathology, allowing the athletic trainer to assess potential systemic illnesses and injuries. For example, Chapter One discusses the process of clinical decision-making, while Chapter Twelve presents evaluation and management algorithms organized by nine common signs and symptoms of systemic pathology (eg, abdominal pain, cough, dyspnea, and fever). Throughout the text, numerous tables and figures summarize complex information. Discussions of medical management for the various illnesses are also noted so that the athletic trainer can gain an awareness of the course of treatment, provide perspective on the athletic trainer's potential role in management of systemic disease, and point out how the treatment (in addition to the illness) may affect participation in physical activity.

Clinical Pathology for Athletic Trainers: Recognizing Systemic Disease provides a unique resource for describing nonorthopedic pathology among athletes and physically active populations. It is intended to be a textbook for athletic training students in accredited educational programs, as well as a reference book for professional athletic trainers. Other health care and fitness professionals, however, who regularly work with athletes and other physically active persons, will find the focused presentation of information to be pertinent and convenient.

Students may find that reading the book chapters in sequential order provides them with the cognitive framework and knowledge necessary to comprehend and integrate the last chapter into practice. Professionals, who may already be familiar with the basic principles and practices of clinical decision-making, can use the last chapter to organize their assessment of suspected nonorthopedic pathology, referencing the detailed descriptions of various diseases and illnesses in the other chapters as necessary to confirm or clarify their differential assessment and clinical decisions. Simply memorizing the algorithms in Chapter Twelve, however, is not a substitute for experience and sound clinical judgment, both of which are only gained by clinical practice. Evaluation of a systemic illness involves the same assessment principles as those used for orthopedic injuries; this book will provide the additional knowledge and skills necessary to do so with confidence.

The information in this text was drawn not only from standard medical reference books, but also from research and reviews published in sports medicine literature over the last 20 years. Readers requiring more information can consult these references to enhance their understanding of any particular topic. Also, every practicing athletic trainer should keep abreast of current medical research and practices, a task made infinitely more easy over the past few years by the omnipresent internet. To this end, many websites are given as resources at the conclusion of each chapter. Some of these sites are essential to the proper appreciation of various illnesses, diseases, and clinical examination procedures. Unfortunately, the internet is by its very nature transient. Hence, although websites come and go, I personally have found the use of the various world wide web search engines invaluable in conducting research for this book. Should some of the sites referenced in this book become obsolete (which will undoubtedly occur), judicious and methodical use of search engines might reveal a multitude of supportive information.

The practice of sports medicine has always involved much more than the evaluation and treatment of musculoskeletal injuries. *Clinical Pathology for Athletic Trainers* supports the expanding utilization of athletic trainers, as witnessed over the last decade, by increasing the basic knowledge and clinical skills available to the profession.

FOREWORD

As the deadline for implementing the 1999 *Competencies in Athletic Training* quickly approaches, program directors across the country, myself included, have been searching for quality resources that adequately address the competencies and proficiencies contained within the new instructional content areas. Finding resources to teach the content areas of pathology of injuries and illnesses and general medical conditions and disabilities have posed a particular challenge. There are numerous athletic training textbooks on the market that address the various aspects of preventing, evaluating, managing, and rehabilitating musculoskeletal injuries; however, few, if any, of these adequately address the recognition and immediate management of general medical conditions and systemic disease. Conversely, there are numerous medical and allied health textbooks that focus on systemic disease. None of these, however, were written specifically for the athletic trainer. Most program directors have been forced to develop their instructional materials for these content areas around several resources, pulling bits and pieces from each one. At last the search for a stand-alone, comprehensive textbook on pathology and general medical conditions is over!

Clinical Pathology for Athletic Trainers: Recognizing Systemic Disease focuses specifically on the nonmusculoskeletal injuries and illnesses that might be encountered by the certified athletic trainer when caring for the physically active. Written by an athletic trainer for the athletic trainer, this text is structured around the required knowledge and skills documented within the 1999 *Competencies in Athletic Training.*

Beginning with a brief review of cellular physiology and the concepts of pathophysiology, this text presents a systematic approach to understanding the common disease processes and their effects on athletes and other physically active individuals. Organized by major body systems, each chapter presents the signs and symptoms of nonmusculoskeletal pathology in a concise, easy-to-read format. The last chapter introduces assessment algorithms for differentiating systemic pathology from musculoskeletal conditions. The algorithms provide a unique approach to helping students synthesize the information presented in previous chapters and develop their decision-making skills. "Red flags" are used to highlight signs and symptoms that would warrant immediate referral to a physician. Beautiful graphics and easy-to-read tables provide readers with a better understanding of the anatomical structures and physiological processes associated with the common systemic pathology.

Athletic training educators will be particularly pleased with the section containing lab activities for teaching auscultation, percussion, and the proper use of the otoscope. Each hands-on lab activity provides students the opportunity to learn, practice, and master the clinical evaluation skills necessary for recognizing general medical conditions.

Clinical Pathology for Athletic Trainers fills an obvious void in the vast array of athletic training textbooks. Mr. O'Connor has done an absolutely wonderful job in presenting potentially complex subject matter in a clear, concise, and easily understood format. This text will make an outstanding addition to the reference library of any athletic trainer—student or professional.

A. Louise Fincher, EdD, ATC, LAT

Chapter One

Principles of Clinical Pathology and Decision-Making

PURPOSES

- Define terminology used to discuss pathology.
- Discuss the role of the athletic trainer with respect to identifying nonmusculoskeletal pathology.
- Review the theoretical and scientific bases of clinical pathology.
- Introduce questions included in a medical history relevant to nonmusculoskeletal pathology.
- Review the behavior and characteristics of symptoms relevant to nonmusculoskeletal pathology.
- Introduce methods of physical examination relevant to nonmusculoskeletal pathology.

INTRODUCTION

Pathology in Sports Medicine and Athletic Training

Pathology, a specialty field of medical science, focuses on the study of biological causes, effects, and processes of disease.[1,2] *Pathogenesis* refers either to the underlying cause of a disease or the actual development of a disease. *Etiology* describes and studies pathogenesis, thus explaining the underlying mechanisms of disease.[2]

Athletic trainers should be aware of all possible origins of injury or illness, particularly for symptoms that are not associated with a specific traumatic incident. Knowledge of pathology and mechanisms of disease will improve clinical decisions. Certain clinical skills, including taking a medical history, performing a physical examination, analyzing clinical information, and making a medical referral, also depend on this knowledge. This textbook reviews the pathogenesis and etiology of many nonmusculoskeletal diseases and pathological conditions.

Signs and Symptoms

A *sign* is an observable indication of pathology, usually discovered during physical examination. A *symptom* is any abnormal function, appearance, or sensation that is experienced by the patient.[2] Thus, signs are objective and measured by the clinician, whereas symptoms are subjective and reported by the patient. Medical conditions often produce signs and symptoms in characteristic patterns.

Each patient's clinical presentation, which is the overall "picture" of signs, symptoms, medical history, and physical examination, can provide clues to possible pathogenesis. This book outlines clinical presentations consistent with nonmusculoskeletal pathology. Standard orthopedic examination and sports medicine texts review how to differentiate between specific injuries of bones, joints, and muscles, and are not discussed here.[3-7]

Diagnosis

The term *diagnosis* refers to the specific injury, illness, disease, or condition a patient has, as determined by medical examination.[2] A clinical diagnosis, which is based on signs and symptoms, medical history, and physical examination, often leads the physician to order laboratory or imaging studies. Analysis of this data results in a differential diagnosis, or the "determination of which of two or more diseases with similar symptoms is the one from which the patient is suffering."[2]

Recognition of Pathology

Most pathological conditions encountered in sports medicine are musculoskeletal in nature. Disorders or disease in any organ or system, however, can occur.[8] Athletic trainers often evaluate persons who have injuries and illnesses before a physician has examined them. Recognizing nonmusculoskeletal medical conditions in such instances allows appropriate intervention or medical referral.[8,9] Allied health care practitioners should be familiar with basic clinical pathology for reasons other than disease recognition. A disease may affect an athlete's ability to participate in sports or other physical activities, or require that certain precautions be taken. Furthermore, a coexisting condition (a medical condition in addition to the primary problem) can complicate recovery from an injury or require treatment modifications.

Theories of Disease and Pathogenesis

Several theories explain the origin and nature of disease. The biomedical model of health and illness attributes disease to abnormal cell, tissue, or organ function in a cause-and-effect relationship.[1] The abnormal function can be caused by anatomical or physiological defects, or by factors such as bacteria and viruses. This book uses the biomedical model to explain pathogenesis for most conditions. Psychosocial theories consider the psychological and social effects on illness and disease.[1] Patients who cannot adapt cognitively or socially to a major injury may be more prone to chronic illness and may not respond to treatment as expected. In addition, psychoemotional stress (eg, academic, financial, social, etc) can confuse the clinical presentation of an illness. Chapter Nine addresses psychological issues in greater detail. Last, genetic factors, such as errors in DNA and RNA replication, can contribute not only to pathogenesis,[1] but also to the effectiveness of the immune system and rate of tissue healing. Genetic and congenital disorders are commonly identified in pediatric patients. Where necessary, the following chapters discuss specific pediatric concerns. It is important to remember that people respond to illness in a variety of ways, depending on individual physical, psychosocial, and genetic factors.

Role of Athletic Trainers in Disease Prevention

The National Athletic Trainers' Association (NATA) identifies injury and illness prevention among physically active persons as a major domain of athletic training practice.[9] Table 1-1 summarizes the three stages of prevention. Primary prevention involves reducing risk factors,[1] which may include nutrition, regular exercise, and removing environmental hazards. Secondary prevention includes early detection of illness or disease and preventing or reversing progression of disease.[1] Tertiary prevention attempts to limit an established disease and restore the highest possible level of function.[1]

Athletic trainers participate in all three stages of prevention. With respect to primary prevention, they identify risk factors, monitor the environment, and counsel athletes. Secondary prevention, such as early detection and appropriate referral, is facilitated by knowledge of clinical pathology. Tertiary prevention provides medical treatment for an injury or illness and continues through return to work or competition.

DIAGNOSTIC REASONING AND
CLINICAL DECISION-MAKING

Diagnostic Reasoning

Medical treatment, as determined and guided by a physician, begins with diagnosis. *Diagnostic reasoning* is the process of differentiating (sorting and interpreting) signs and symptoms by a physician to arrive at a diagnosis. A diagnosis leads to actions such as administration of medications, surgery, referral to medical specialists, or referral to allied health

Table 1-1
STAGES OF DISEASE PREVENTION

Stage	Goals	Interventions
Primary	Reduce risk factors	Nutrition, exercise, monitoring environmental risks, prevention, and education programs
Secondary	Early detection, early intervention, inhibit progression of disease	Regular medical checkups, self-examination, and early medical treatment
Tertiary	Limit established disease	Supportive and restorative medical treatment

services. Diagnostic processes include triage (determining the urgency of a medical condition), medical history, physical examination, laboratory tests, and imaging studies.[10]

Clinical Decision-Making

Athletic trainers do not make medical diagnoses. They instead use clinical decision-making, a process similar to diagnostic reasoning. *Clinical decision-making* determines the best course of action for a particular patient, leading to processes such as first aid, emergency transport, rehabilitation, reassessment, modification of treatment, or referral to other health care specialists. Recognizing characteristic patterns of signs and symptoms can suggest the potential pathogenesis and help to determine a course of action.

Table 1-2 compares diagnostic reasoning and clinical decision-making. The remainder of this chapter discusses the information used to make clinical decisions. This information is collected from the medical history, signs and symptoms, and the physical examination.

MEDICAL HISTORY

A *medical history* is "an account of the events," previous and current, related to a patient's state of health.[10] All injured athletes require a medical history. The scope and extent of the history, however, should be appropriate to the situation. For instance, primary assessment of a traumatic injury need not include a full medical history. A person who reports vague or unusual symptoms while undergoing assessment in an outpatient clinic, however, needs more extensive questioning.[11]

Taking a Medical History

Upon first interaction with an injured or ill person, the athletic trainer collects components of the medical history, as listed in Table 1-3.[10,12,13] Details reported by the patient are recorded if they are potentially relevant to subsequent physical examination, treatment, or outcome. Initiating treatment without taking a medical history is not appropriate, except perhaps in an emergency. Table 1-4 gives the purposes of the medical history.

Table 1-2

CLINICAL DECISION-MAKING VERSUS DIAGNOSTIC REASONING

	Clinical Decision-Making	Diagnostic Reasoning
Clinician	Athletic trainer	Physician
Goals	Determine the potential nature of the disorder and the course of action	Determine a medical diagnosis and course of medical treatment
Processes	History, physical exam, reassessment (evaluate progress)	History, physical exam, form hypothesis, confirm hypothesis (with medical laboratory and imaging)
Results	Emergency transport, first aid, rehabilitation, referral to health care specialists, modify treatment	Medication, surgery, referral to health care specialists

Table 1-3

COMPONENTS OF A MEDICAL HISTORY

- Chief complaint
- Description and course of present illness
- Personal medical history
- Family medical history
- Review of systems

A proper medical history focuses on the patient's issues and establishes an immediate rapport (trust) between the clinician and the patient.[11] Conducting a medical history requires practice to obtain complete, correct, and honest information. This information begins to build the patient's clinical presentation.

Participants in organized athletics usually receive a preparticipation examination. This includes a physical screening examination, a survey of personal and family medical history, and a review of systems. This survey-type medical history can identify existing pathology that prevents or limits participation in specific sports. This preliminary medical record should be consulted when evaluating injuries and illnesses incurred during the season. In addition to traditional athletic settings, athletic trainers also work in clinics and as contract employees at athletic events. In these situations, the athletic trainer is unfamiliar with the patient so the entire medical history is collected during initial injury assessment.

Chief Complaints

The *chief complaints* are symptoms that cause a patient to seek medical attention.[10] Pain in a particular body segment is often one of the chief complaints. Some patients are also concerned with disability (inability to perform) in sport, work, or social-familial duties. The ath-

---

Table 1-4

PURPOSE OF A MEDICAL HISTORY

- Determine potential pathogenesis
- Identify coexisting conditions
- Determine the extent of the injury or illness
- Identify contraindications to treatment

Table 1-5

HISTORY OF PRESENT ILLNESS

- When did your condition start?
- What makes your condition better? What makes it worse?
- Is your condition better or worse in the morning or at night?
- Is your condition better or worse with breathing, urination, eating, excitement, stress, rest, or certain body positions?
- Have you had x-rays, MRIs, or CT scans for this condition?
- What treatment have you received for this condition?
- Is your condition getting better, getting worse, or not changing either way?
- Have you ever had any condition like this before?
- Is there anything else I need to know about you or your condition?

---

letic trainer uses the chief complaints to focus the assessment in order to evaluate the effects of injury or illness, as baseline indicators with which to monitor recovery, and to tend to the patient's goals.

Description and Course of Present Illness

The core of the history-taking process is the history of present illness. This includes the patient's description of onset of symptoms, progression of symptoms since onset, and the nature of the problem. Table 1-5 lists some common questions asked during the history of the present illness. Details about the onset and presence of symptoms, as well as how those symptoms have changed in intensity, frequency, or duration, are important. Inquiring whether the condition is "getting better, not changing, or getting worse" indicates the progression of the disease. The patient should rate his or her symptoms numerically using visual or verbal analog scales (Figure 1-1), which can be repeated each day to assess recovery. At the conclusion of the history of present illness, the clinician should have a good idea about the patient's condition. For instance, how did it begin and how has it changed? What are the frequency, intensity, and duration of symptoms? And what makes the condition better or worse?

Personal and Family Medical History

The personal medical history and family medical history review previous significant medical conditions or illnesses experienced by the patient and immediate family members (Table 1-6). Some responses lead to more specific questions, particularly since patients may not con-

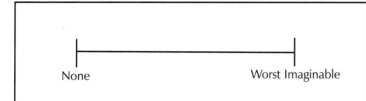

Figure 1-1. 100-mm visual analog scale.

None   Worst Imaginable

Instructions: mark on the line to indicate how much pain you are having.

Table 1-6

PAST AND FAMILY MEDICAL HISTORY

heart disease	kidney disease	headaches	anemia
stroke	breathing problems	depression	substance abuse
digestive problems	nerve problems	high blood	
arthritis	diabetes	pressure	
cancer	liver disease	recurrent infections	

* Have you or any immediate family member had any of the above major health problems?
* How is your current health?
* Do you currently have any other injuries or medical conditions?
* Have you ever been admitted to a hospital?
* Have you ever had surgery?

sider "minor" surgeries or health problems to be relevant to their present condition. A coexisting condition may require the athletic trainer to modify assessment or treatment techniques. A family history of systemic disease may be relevant if clinical presentation suggests similar systemic pathology.

Review of Systems

The review of systems screens for major organ system disease by asking about specific symptoms (Table 1-7). This can be done by interview or questionnaire. When any of these symptoms are present, more specific questions relative to the respective systems are indicated, as addressed in subsequent chapters.[14]

Medical Tests

Physicians use radiographs (x-rays), magnetic resonance imaging (MRI), laboratory tests (eg, blood, urinalysis), and many other medical tests to make a diagnosis. If and when medical tests for the current condition have been performed should be determined.[13] In addition, medications for all current and coexisting medical conditions should be documented. Many medications have side effects or require treatment precautions. The NATA Research and Education Foundation provides an excellent review of pharmacology.[15,16]

Table 1-7

REVIEW OF SYSTEMS BY SYMPTOM

General Systemic Symptoms	Potential System of Origin
Fever, chills, sweats	Infection or immune system cancer
Severe night pain	Cancer, cardiovascular, gastrointestinal
Unexplained weight change	Gastrointestinal, metabolic, depression, eating disorder, infection, cancer
Unusual fatigue, malaise	Depression, infection, endocrine, diabetes, anemia, rheumatoid arthritis, eating disorder, cancer
Key System-Specific Symptoms	
Chest pain or palpitations	Cardiovascular
Shortness of breath	Cardiovascular, pulmonary
Dizziness, light-headedness, fainting	Cardiovascular, medications, metabolic
Nausea, vomiting	Gastrointestinal, pregnancy, cancer, drug toxicity
Loss of control of bowels (diarrhea)	Gastrointestinal
Difficulty, bleeding, or pain while urinating	Urogenital, infection
Sexual function problems	Urogenital, neurological, psychological
Visual disturbances	Neurological, cardiovascular
Numbness, weakness, burning, tingling	Neurological
Difficulty swallowing, hoarseness	Neurological, gastrointestinal, neoplasm

General Health Questions

Poor recent health may indicate occult (undetected) pathology or progression of a known medical condition. Thus, questions related to the person's current health may be necessary (Table 1-8). Men and women may also need screening questions relative to their respective reproductive systems (see Chapter Six). Sport, work environment, or regular physical activity (or inactivity) may be related to pathogenesis, treatment, prognosis (predicted outcome of

---

Table 1-8

RECENT GENERAL HEALTH STATUS

- Have you lost more than 5 to 10 lbs in the last month?
- What regular physical stresses does your job involve?

sitting	walking	climbing
desk work	lifting	exposure to chemicals
standing	small equipment	
large equipment	bending	

- Are you on a diet?
- Do you use any tobacco products?
- How much alcohol do you drink in a week?
- How many caffeinated drinks do you have in a day?

---

disease), and recovery. Age, gender, race, or occupation may also be relevant to pathogenesis.[11] Important social information to collect includes regular physical stresses (eg, sitting, driving, lifting), psychoemotional stress, exposure to toxins (including smoke, alcohol, caffeine, and drugs), and usual schedule (ie, does the person have time to "fit in" good nutrition, medical treatment, appointments, etc).[11]

Interpretation of the Medical History

Information collected in the medical history directs the subsequent physical examination. In the chapters that follow, symptom patterns relevant to systemic pathology will be presented. Components of the physical examination, which is used to gain further information and complete the clinical presentation, will be reviewed. A complete clinical presentation assists clinical decision-making.

SYMPTOMS

Behavior and Characteristics

Qualities of various symptoms can reveal the nature of the disorder.[11] Table 1-9 compares qualities of systemic (nonmusculoskeletal) and musculoskeletal symptoms. Pain of systemic origin is usually constant, unchanged by movement or posture, most intense at night, and present during function of the affected system(s). Musculoskeletal pain is usually intermittent, changed by body position or posture, decreased at night, and is unaffected by function of the internal organ system. Table 1-10 lists certain words patients may use to describe symptoms of pathology in various body systems.

Anatomical location of symptoms also provides additional clues. The patient can either draw his or her symptom pattern on a body diagram (Figure 1-2) or simply point to his or her symptomatic areas. Each organ and system has a characteristic referral pattern, each of which

Table 1-9

CHARACTER AND BEHAVIOR OF SYSTEMIC AND MUSCULOSKELETAL SYMPTOMS

Systemic	Musculoskeletal
Constant	Intermittent
No change with movement or posture	Consistent change with movement or posture
No change or worse at rest	Relief with rest
Worse at night	Relief at night
Worse with organ function	Unaffected by organ function

Table 1-10

PAIN DESCRIPTORS AND POSSIBLE SYSTEMIC ORIGIN OF PATHOLOGY

System	Descriptors
Vascular	Pulsing, throbbing, pounding, cramping, quivering
Neurogenic	Shooting, stabbing, drilling, sharp, cutting, pinching, pressing, pulling, burning, tingling, stinging
Musculoskeletal	Dull, sore, hurting, aching, heavy
Emotional lability (psychoemotional)	Splitting, exhausting, sickening, cruel, vicious, killing, unbearable, radiating, tight, cold, nagging

are presented in subsequent chapters. Symptoms that match these visceral (organ) patterns should prompt investigation for other signs.

Acute and Chronic

The term *acute pain* describes pain of sudden onset with high intensity and relatively short duration (hours or days). *Chronic pain* appears insidiously (very gradually), with lower intensity and a much longer duration (weeks or months). Acute pain without trauma, or chronic pain that returns in predictable cycles or progresses in intensity, suggests systemic pathology.

Local and Referred

Local pain stays in a specific region or area of the body. *Referred pain*, however, occurs in a region distal to the damaged tissue. Although referred pain can occur with certain musculoskeletal injuries, it may also indicate systemic pathology.

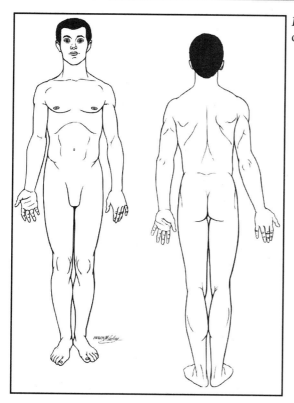

Figure 1-2. Body diagram for location of pain or other symptoms.

Constant and Intermittent

Constant pain is always present, although the intensity may vary over time. Patients describe *intermittent pain* as something that "comes and goes." With either type, if intensity varies with a certain movement or body position, an acute musculoskeletal injury may be suspected. Conversely, if intensity increases at night, with organ function (eg, digestion, urination), or does not change at all, the pain may be systemic in origin.

Causes of Pain

Mechanical, chemical, and perceptual mechanisms cause different types of pain, although they can occur in combination with one another.

Mechanical Pain

Anatomical structures under physical stress produce *mechanical pain*. Most commonly, musculoskeletal injuries cause this type of pain. Mechanical pain is intermittent, related to movement or position, and relieved by removing the offending stress. Mechanical pain appears only in the injured structure.

Chemical Pain

Biochemical substances released with tissue injury produce *chemical pain*. These substances irritate innervated tissues and cause inflammation, as briefly reviewed in Chapter Two. Chemical pain is constant, although intensity may change. This type of pain cannot be relieved by movement or position, although it may be increased by them. Medication near-

Figure 1-3. Dermatomal patterns.

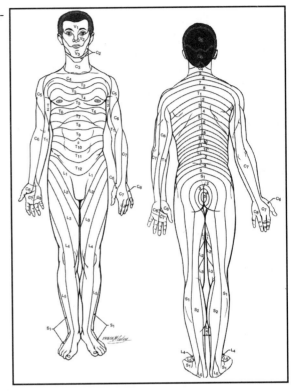

ly always decreases chemical pain. Chemical pain is poorly localized and refers to other locations if a nerve or adjacent anatomical structures are affected.

Perceptual Pain

Pain itself is a perception, so all types of pain have perceptual components. Individual
response to pain is a product of previous cultural, social, and personal experiences. It is also
possible for the physical (mechanical and chemical) origin of pain to be removed, but the
perception of pain to remain. This indicates a strong psychological or social contribution to
the condition. If an athletic trainer recognizes this situation, he or she should refer the person appropriately and support the prescribed treatment.

Pain-Generating Tissues

Different tissues also produce different types of pain, each of which can be present simultaneously. Skin and superficial subcutaneous tissues generate cutaneous pain, localized to the
area of tissue damage. Deep somatic pain originates in bones, nerves, muscles, tendons, ligaments, arteries, or joints. Deep somatic pain often refers to cutaneous sites that correspond
to the same spinal level, or dermatome, as the affected tissue. It may cause autonomic reactions such as sweating, pallor, nausea, and syncope. The internal organs of the cardiovascular, hematological, pulmonary, digestive, urogenital, endocrine, and reproductive systems
can produce visceral pain. Visceral pain receptors (nociceptors) relay a diffuse signal that
refers to associated dermatomes, as shown in Figure 1-3. This type of pain also produces a
deep, gnawing ache in the thorax or abdomen.

Table 1-11

SYMPTOMS REQUIRING URGENT REFERRAL TO A PHYSICIAN: RED FLAGS

- Constant pain
- Heart palpitations/flutter
- Fainting (syncope)
- Night pain or night sweats
- Difficult or painful swallowing
- Visual problems
- Unexplained weight loss
- Insomnia
- Incapacitating pain

- Severe dyspnea
- Recurrent nausea, vomiting
- Pulsating or severe cramping pain (colic)
- Difficult or painful urination
- Blood in the urine
- Severe or progressive dizziness
- Malaise, fatigue

Red Flags

Certain signs and symptoms alert the athletic trainer to serious pathology (Table 1-11). These red flags require immediate medical attention. Some red flags are obvious emergencies (eg, loss of consciousness, breathing, or circulation), but others, such as recurrent fevers, pain at night, malaise, unexplained weight loss, and insomnia, may be discovered during the medical history or physical examination. Symptoms that are not well localized, have no injury associated with onset, have been relentlessly worsening, and are unaffected by standard treatments are also not likely to be caused by a musculoskeletal condition.

PHYSICAL EXAMINATION TECHNIQUES: DIFFERENTIATING NORMAL AND ABNORMAL RESPONSES

Physical examination for systemic pathology has several components (Table 1-12). The physical examination process is modified according to suspected pathogenesis, the patient's symptoms, and urgency of the patient's condition.

Inspection

Inspection involves observing of general appearance, skin, hair, and nails, obvious deformities, use of assistive devices or supports, behavior, gait, and coordination. Many systemic conditions cause "classic" signs of disease that can be observed during this phase of examination.

Vital Signs

The *vital signs* are heart rate, respiration rate, blood pressure, and body temperature. Vital signs should be assessed in emergencies and when systemic symptoms (see Table 1-7) are reported. If a patient's medical history includes hypertension, cardiac pathology, recent infection, chronic illness, or cancer, vital signs should be recorded to indicate present health status and provide a baseline to monitor health status throughout treatment.

> Table 1-12
> # COMPONENTS OF THE PHYSICAL EXAMINATION
> - Inspection/observation
> - Vital signs
> - Percussion
> - Palpation
> - Smell/odor
> - Auscultation
> - Neurological exam

Percussion and Palpation

Percussion (striking to cause vibration) over the vertebrae or other bones may increase pain of fractures or bone tumors. Percussion over the thorax and abdomen vibrates internal organs and can detect pathology in a similar manner. Superficial *palpation* (manual touch or manipulation) can assess skin temperature, texture, moisture, and turgidity (stiffness), and is used to examine lymph nodes and vascular pulses. Detection of abnormal masses, abdominal rigidity (see Chapter Five), and tenderness is achieved through deep palpation.

Auscultation

Auscultation is performed with an instrument called a stethoscope to examine cardiac, pulmonary, vascular, abdominal, and bowel sounds. Auscultation technique will be discussed in several of the following chapters.

Smell

Unusual odor of the breath or perspiration suggests expulsion of metabolic substances, which can indicate pathology, poisoning, or drug abuse. Foul-smelling sputum or other body fluids can indicate infection or endocrine malfunction.

Neurological Screening Exam

Any patient reporting radiating pain, sensory abnormalities, weakness, or recent head injury should receive a neurological screening examination of the cranial nerves, reflexes, sensation, and motor function.

Cranial Nerves and Reflexes

Cranial nerves control smell, vision and eye control, facial sensation, facial motor control, hearing, swallowing, gag reflex, shoulder blade elevation, and tongue control. Cranial nerve testing is reviewed in Chapter Eight.

The deep tendon *reflexes* include biceps (C5), brachioradialis (C6), triceps (C7), patella (L2-4), and ankle (S1).[17] Lab Activity 1 outlines reflex testing. The Babinski sign is an abnormal reflex that appears when the motor tracts descending from the brain are disrupted, which occurs with spinal cord or severe head injuries.

Table 1-13
MYOTOMAL DISTRIBUTION

Nerve Root	Muscles	
C1	Captial rotators	Head rotation
C2	None	Sensory only (occiput)
C3 to C4	Levator scapulae	Shoulder elevation (with CN XI)
C5	Biceps	Elbow flexion
C6	Extensor carpi radialis Brevis/longus	Wrist extension
C7	Triceps	Elbow extension
C8	Abductor pollicis longus/brevis	Thumb abduction
T1	Interossei of the hand	Abduction of fingers (squeezing together)
T2 to T12	Segmental intercostals	Inhalation, exhalation
L1 to L2	Psoas major	Hip flexion
L2 to L4	Quadriceps	Knee extension
L4	Anterior tibialis	Ankle dorsiflexion
L5	Extensor hallicus longus	Great toe extension (dorsiflexion)
S1	Peroneals	Ankle eversion
S1 to 2	Gastrocnemius	Ankle plantarflexion

Sensory Testing

Sensation should be tested bilaterally along dermatomal and peripheral nerve distributions. Light touch, which is transmitted up both halves of the spinal cord, is tested first. If impairments are found, sharp (or temperature) and vibration senses may also be tested to examine the opposite (contralateral) and same side (ipsilateral) spinal cord columns, respectively.

Motor Testing

Gross testing of muscle strength may be done manually to differentiate between myotomal (nerve root), peripheral nerve, or muscle lesions. Injured or inflamed nerve roots produce weakness in many associated muscles (Table 1-13). Peripheral nerve damage affects only the few muscles supplied by that nerve. Traumatic muscle injuries weaken only one specific muscle. Nerve injuries may not cause significant pain but do cause substantial weakness. Muscle injuries are usually both weak and painful. Physician referral is indicated with any sign of new or progressive neurological compromise.

SUMMARY

Athletic trainers use clinical decision-making to evaluate possible pathogenesis. This process includes taking a medical history, evaluating symptom patterns, and performing a physical examination. The medical history provides information regarding onset of the condition, previous similar problems, and the nature and course of the illness. The quality, behavior, characteristics, and description of symptoms can identify potential systemic pathology. The physical examination identifies signs that confirm the history and reported symptoms and completes the clinical presentation. In the next chapter, basic pathophysiology of the organs and systems of the body is discussed.

RESOURCES

General Medical References

- atlife.com contains a search engine to thousands of medical sites and information. www.atlife.com/life
- Dr.Koop.com; former US Surgeon General Dr. CE Koop's online medical encyclopedia. www.drkoop.com/conditions/ency
- Emedicine.com online medical textbooks, including: dermatology, emergency medicine and family health, neurology, pediatrics, orthopedics, and sports medicine. www.emedicine.com/cgi-shl/foxweb.exe/onlinebooks@d:/em/ga
- Gray's Anatomy online. www.bartleby.com/107
- Medicalstudent.com full-text manuals for various medical conditions and the basic medical sciences. www.medicalstudent.com
- Medline plus (National Library of Medicine) medical encyclopedia. medlineplus.adam.com
- The Merck Manual online; a searchable, authoritative medical reference containing information on examination, etiology, signs and symptoms, medical testing, differential diagnoses, medical treatment, and prognosis for thousands of diseases and medical conditions. www.merck.com/pubs/mmanual
- The Michigan Electronic Library's list of online health and medical dictionaries and glossaries. mel.lib.mi.us/health/health-dictionaries.html
- oso.com illustrated medical encyclopedia. www.oso.com/shared/health/adam_index.html
- United States Navy general medical officer manual. www.vnh.org/GMO/01Contents.html
- Yahoo directory, includes over 1300 active links to information about specific diseases. dir.yahoo.com/Health/Diseases_and_Conditions

Pharmacology

- atlife.com pharmacology site. www.atpharmacology.com/pharm
- PharmInfoNet glossary of pharmaceutical and medical terminology. pharminfo.com/pia_glos.html

Physical Examination Techniques

- Loyola University Medical Education Network's page on physical exam techniques. www.meddean.luc.edu/lumen/meded/medicine/pulmonar/pd/contents.htm

REFERENCES

1. Goodman CC. Introduction to concepts of pathology. In: Goodman CC, Boissonnault WG, eds. *Pathology: Implications for the Physical Therapist.* Philadelphia, Pa: WB Saunders Company; 1998:3-8.

2. Hensyl WR, ed. *Stedman's Pocket Medical Dictionary.* Baltimore, Md: Williams & Wilkins; 1987.

3. Anderson MK, Hall SJ. *Sports Injury Management.* 2nd ed. Philadelphia, Pa: Lippincott Williams & Wilkins; 2000.

4. Arnheim DD, Prentice WE. *Principles of Athletic Training.* 8th ed. St. Louis, Mo: Mosby-Year Book; 1993.

5. Hertling D, Kessler RM. *Management of Common Musculoskeletal Disorders.* 2nd ed. Philadelphia, Pa: JB Lippincott Company; 1990.

6. Magee DJ. *Orthopedic Physical Assessment.* 2nd ed. Philadelphia, Pa: WB Saunders Company; 1992.

7. Saunders HD, Woerman AL. *Evaluation, Treatment, and Prevention of Musculoskeletal Disorders.* Bloomington, Minn: Educational Opportunities; 1985.

8. Arnheim DD, Prentice WE. Other health conditions related to sports. In: Arnheim DD, Prentice WE, eds. *Principles of Athletic Training.* 8th ed. St. Louis, Mo: Mosby-Year Book; 1993:796-819.

9. National Athletic Trainers' Association Board of Certification. *1999 NATABOC Role Delineation Study.* Omaha, Neb: National Athletic Trainers' Association Board of Certification Inc; 1999.

10. DeGowin RL, Brown DD. *DeGowin's Diagnostic Examination.* 7th ed. New York: McGraw-Hill; 2000.

11. Bickley LS, Hoekelman RA. *Bates' Guide to Physical Examination and History Taking.* 7th ed. Philadelphia, Pa: Lippincott Williams & Wilkins; 1999.

12. Boissonnault WG, Janos SC. Screening for medical disease: physical therapy assessment and treatment principles. In: Boissonnault WG, ed. *Examination in Physical Therapy Practice: Screening for Medical Disease.* New York: Churchill Livingstone; 1995:1-30.

13. Goodman CC, Snyder TEK. Introduction to the interviewing process. In: Goodman CC, Snyder TEK, eds. *Differential Diagnosis in Physical Therapy: Musculoskeletal and Systemic Conditions.* 3rd ed. Philadelphia, Pa: WB Saunders Company; 2000:37-87.

14. Goodman CC, Snyder TEK. Introduction to differential screening in physical therapy. In: Goodman CC, Snyder TEK, eds. *Differential Diagnosis in Physical Therapy: Musculoskeletal and Systemic Conditions.* 3rd ed. Philadelphia, Pa: WB Saunders Company; 2000:1-36.

15. National Athletic Trainers' Association. *Pharmacology for Athletic Trainers: Therapeutic Medications.* Champaign, Ill: Human Kinetics; 1997.

16. National Athletic Trainers' Association. *Pharmacology for Athletic Trainers: Performance Enhancement and Social Drugs.* Champaign, Ill: Human Kinetics; 1997.

17. Hoppenfeld S. *Physical Examination of the Spine and Extremities.* Norwalk, Conn: Appleton & Lange; 1976.

Chapter Two

Pathophysiology

PURPOSES

- Describe cellular components and their functions.
- Discuss the inflammatory process.
- Review pathophysiology by tissue type.
- Describe cellular adaptations to disease.
- Explain the concept of homeostasis.
- Explain cellular adaptation and regulatory mechanisms in response to disease.

INTRODUCTION

This chapter will not replace formal study and understanding of normal cell structure and physiology. It briefly reviews normal physiology and introduces the concepts of pathophysiology (physiology of disease). These topics provide a basis for discussing systemic pathology in subsequent chapters. Many clinical and cellular pathophysiology textbooks are available should the reader desire greater detail on any particular topic.[1-5]

Homeostasis

Homeostasis involves many processes that regulate the complex biochemical equilibrium within the body. These mechanisms constantly restore fluid, chemical, and energy balance in cells, tissues, organs, and systems of the body.[1,6] As part of normal function, the biological balance in these systems is constantly disturbed and restored. For example, blood glucose level increases after eating a meal. In response, cells in the pancreas release insulin, a hormone that moves glucose from the blood to the liver and muscles. Once the blood glucose level has returned to normal, insulin secretion decreases to prevent blood glucose levels from becoming too low. These normal stimulus-response cycles are necessary to maintain health.

This healthy state, however, is somewhat specific to each individual. Thus, "normal" values for chemical and functional indicators (eg, blood test results and vital signs) are usually described as a range that depends on age, gender, physical fitness, and genetic factors. In addition, these values may exceed "normal" range to maintain organ-system function in response to extreme internal and external demands. For instance, persons living in very high altitudes have a significantly higher number of circulating red blood cells since the concentration of atmospheric oxygen is much lower than at sea level. This increase in red blood cell volume allows the blood to hold an adequate amount of oxygen even though less oxygen is available in the atmosphere.

Pathophysiology

Many pathological processes disrupt the processes of homeostasis, causing a deviation from the normal, balanced biochemical state. *Pathophysiology* describes the cellular mechanisms of disease and their systemic (functional) consequences.[1] Similar to "normal" values, signs and symptoms of pathology usually follow general patterns depending on the affected systems but may vary from person to person. Understanding the normal physiology and the independent and interrelated functions of the body's organ systems augments the discussion of the effects of disease. Study of physiology begins with the basic unit of the body's tissues: the cell.

The Cell

All living cells, regardless of the tissue they comprise, contains many structures, including cytoplasm, a nucleus, lysosomes, mitochondria, and a cell membrane, each of which serves a particular purpose (Table 2-1).[6] Each cell includes genetic material, energy sources, and enzymes. Cells can be damaged by physical trauma; exposure to toxins; infection; genetic abnormalities (affecting cell structure or cell division); deprivation of nutrients, water, or oxygen (metabolic); or combinations of these factors.[1,4] Disease or injury damages one or more cell structures, causing impairment of tissue and organ function, which in turn affects func-

Table 2-1

CELL STRUCTURES AND THEIR FUNCTIONS

Structure	Function
Nucleus	Contains genetic material of the cell (DNA and RNA) Controls cell division and synthesis of protein
Cytoplasm	Provides internal fluid environment of the cell Supports all internal cell structures
Lysosomes	Contains catabolic enzymes within the cell Disposes of cell waste and foreign substances
Mitochondria	Converts carbohydrate, protein, and fat to ATP (energy)
Cell membrane	Consists of complex semipermeable phospholipid and protein structures Provides the physical border of the cell Excludes or exchanges substances between the internal and external environment of the cell

tion of the associated system or systems. Cells of other tissues and organs can be affected as the consequence of disease spread to surrounding tissues. Some effects of cell damage initiate responses that attempt to limit the disease process, initiate cell repair, and restore homeostasis.

Once cell damage occurs, the cell either adapts or dies. Adaptation occurs if the cell can access internal resources to maintain function of the nucleus and begin repair.[1,4] Adaptation, however, may affect the normal function of the cell, leading to subsequent problems in the tissue or organ. Cells may also respond to environmental factors by adapting before cell damage occurs.

Cells adapt in several ways.[1] First, they can shrink in response to decreased metabolic demands, a process called *atrophy*, or grow in response to increased demands, called *hypertrophy*. Atrophy is generally caused by disuse (eg, injury or immobilization) or impaired cellular metabolism (eg, malnutrition). Hypertrophy, conversely, increases cell size to meet increased metabolic or physical demands (eg, weight lifting). Atrophic or hypertrophic cells are underactive or overactive, respectively, with accompanying physiological consequences. Aging is a type of atrophic cellular adaptation caused by multiple factors, including cell damage caused by internal (metabolic) and external toxic exposures accumulated over a lifetime.

Cells may also adapt by changing in number, type, or morphology (structure). Hyperplasia increases the number of cells in a given tissue without changing the rate of cell division or cell function. This occurs as an adaptation to chronic increased metabolic demands, genetic abnormalities, or hormonal imbalances. Metaplasia replaces cells of one type with cells of another type, often in response to physical or chemical irritants. These "new" cells do not changes rate of division or function, but may change the relative proportion of one cell type to another within a particular tissue.

When cells adapt by changing to an abnormal cell type, increasing the rate of division, and increasing in number, *dysplasia* has occurred. Dysplasia, similar to metaplasia except producing abnormal cells, can be caused by chronic irritation or a malfunction in DNA replication. Formation of neoplasms, or tumors, involve dysplasia. Malignant (severely invasive) dysplasia produces neoplasms in a process called cancer (rapid proliferation of undifferentiated cells, or nonspecific cell types). Cell death, or necrosis, occurs when cell resources cannot meet the metabolic (ie, oxygen and energy) demands of the nucleus. A large number of dead cells impairs organ function, thus disabling the associated body system. Cell necrosis can lead to disease or death of the organism.

Most normal cellular adaptations, such as callus formation (hyperplasia) or menstruation (hyperplasia and metaplasia), are temporary physiological responses that restore homeostasis. Other adaptations or cell damage, however, produce general chemical and physical responses that occur to repair tissue structure or function. An example of such a general response is inflammation. Other effects are caused by tissue-specific adaptations. The general and specific effects may impair organ function, thus becoming pathological and causing signs and symptoms.

Inflammation

System-specific signs and symptoms will be outlined in subsequent chapters when describing pathological conditions. Signs and symptoms of the general inflammatory response, however, are discussed here. Understanding the cellular inflammatory response is important. Every tissue of the body responds to cellular injury or infection with *inflammation*. The inflammatory response can either be limited only to the affected tissue, producing localized symptoms, or be generalized, causing "systemic" symptoms (see Table 1-7). Consequently, many signs and symptoms are common to pathology that affects multiple systems.

Acute Inflammation

Damaged cells immediately release chemicals (eg, histamine, bradykinin, prostaglandin) that cause local capillaries to dilate and become permeable. This increases blood flow to the area and allows proteins and plasma fluid to enter the interstitial space (between cells).[1] Proteins in the blood interact with fibrin and begin to form a collagen clot at the damaged site. The chemicals released by the damaged cells also attract leukocytes from the blood. Several types of leukocytes are activated, some acting as phagocytes and others that prolong the inflammatory response. Phagocytes chemically dissolve and absorb damaged cell structures, invading microbes, and foreign debris.

As inflammation continues, excess interstitial fluid causes a rise in tissue pressure relative to pressure in the capillaries. Blood flow in the area consequently decreases, producing ischemic damage in otherwise healthy cells, thus increasing tissue damage. This secondary tissue damage is greatest near the site of primary cell injury.

These mechanisms cause the characteristic signs and symptoms of inflammation. Pain results from tissue damage (primary and secondary), chemical mediators, and ischemia. Swelling, erythema (redness), and heat are effects of increased regional blood flow and plasma fluid in the interstitial space. Ecchymosis (dark red, blue, or black discoloration) from red blood cells in the tissues may occur. Pain causes local muscle spasm to guard the damaged tissue, thus causing loss of movement and function. The acute phase of inflammation somewhat depends on the extent of cellular damage but generally lasts from 48 to 72 hours.

Chronic Inflammation

Chronic inflammation, which can also occur in any tissue, is usually a result of long-standing or repetitive chemical (internal metabolic products or external toxins) irritation or mechanical stress. Chronic inflammation is potentially very destructive to the cells and tissues since the biochemical action and leukocyte activity is prolonged. In addition, chronic inflammation produces much more fibrin and collagen to protect the undamaged tissue or isolate the offending substance. Thus, chronic inflammation may actually prevent or inhibit tissue healing. The signs and symptoms are the same as acute inflammation but somewhat less intense. Chronic inflammation produces aching pain, pitting edema (as the fluid and proteins in the interstitial space consolidate), mild to moderate muscle spasms, and increased local tissue temperature. Chronic inflammation persists until the cause of cellular damage is removed.

Infection

The response to infection (an invasion of microorganisms; see Chapter Nine) is essentially a specialized inflammatory response. Cell damage caused by the infectious organism causes an inflammatory response, as outlined above. In addition, activation of the immune system can also stimulate a generalized inflammatory response. This response is much more widespread than occurs with a local tissue wound. Activated leukocytes in the blood affect neurons in the medulla, which cause an increase in the overall temperature of the body. Involuntary shivering (chills), widespread vasoconstriction, and lying down and flexing the body all occur to increase body temperature to a new level. This process is called *fever*.

The presence of fever significantly increases metabolic demands of the body's cells. This causes hyperpnea (rapid respiration) and tachycardia (rapid heart rate), as well as breakdown (catabolism) of muscle and other tissues to obtain energy. Interestingly, fat is not utilized in this process. The effects of fever are unusual fatigue, malaise (feeling bad), weakness, and loss of appetite. Once the microorganism has been eliminated, the fever "breaks." To reduce body temperature, the person exhibits diaphoresis (sweating), lethargy (extreme drowsiness), and extension of the body in supine. In addition, appetite returns to replace energy stores that were drained during the course of the fever. The duration of fever depends on the virulence (aggressiveness) of the infection.

CELLULAR PHYSIOLOGY AND PATHOPHYSIOLOGY: RESPONSE TO CELLULAR DAMAGE

Bone

Normal Morphology and Physiology

Bone provides a framework for the body, levers for muscle, and protection for internal organs (heart, lungs, kidneys, liver, spleen, brain, and spinal cord). Mature bone cells are called osteocytes, which are produced by osteoblasts and reabsorbed by osteoclasts.[1] Each bone is covered by periosteum, an innervated and vascular structure that provides nutrition to the cortical (compact) bone. Cancellous (spongy) bone has its own blood supply and contains the bone marrow. Bone marrow is either yellow (fatty) or red. The red marrow, a critical organ, produces blood cells.[1] In children, most bones contain red marrow, whereas adults have red marrow only in the flat bones (cranium, ribs, pelvis, vertebrae).[1]

Bones articulate to form joints. Joint surfaces are covered with articular cartilage, which decreases the friction between the opposing bones. Articular cartilage is avascular, has no nervous supply, and has very few chondrocytes (living cartilage cells) within its tissue.

Pathological Processes

Fracture—physical damage to a bone—can occur across an entire bone, involving both cortical and cancellous bone, or occur only in the cortical bone (eg, greenstick and stress fractures). A fracture that penetrates the skin, called an "open" fracture, is particularly prone to infection. Bone infection causes osteomyelitis (inflammation of bone and marrow; see Chapter Nine), which destroys normal bone cells and deforms the bone. Many genetic and metabolic abnormalities of bone, such as osteogenesis imperfecta and osteoporosis, can produce severe deformity and disability. Toxic damage, such as exposure to high-dosage radiation, is another possible source of pathology. Articular cartilage can be damaged by physical trauma (osteochondritis dissecans), inflammation (osteoarthritis, rheumatoid arthritis), or infection.

Response to Disease or Injury

Fractured bone can heal given the appropriate environment (alignment and approximation of bone ends, stability, sterility, and nutrition).[1] Fracture healing takes place in several stages.[1] The first is a local inflammatory response, including bleeding (hematoma formation) and muscle guarding. As the hematoma resolves and a fibrin clot forms, osteoblast activity increases to produce new bone cells. Fibrocartilage forms around the fracture and is then gradually replaced by a bony callus or mass of osteocytes in various stages of formation. Once the bony callus is complete, the bone is stable and can bear weight. This process takes approximately 4 to 6 weeks in children and 8 to 12 weeks in adults.[1] For 1 to 2 years following the fracture, the bone remodels in response to the demands placed upon it.

Bone infections heal by a similar mechanism as long as the infection is eliminated, which often involves surgical resection and stabilization. Genetic and metabolic bone disorders, such as osteogenesis imperfecta or osteoporosis (see Chapter Seven), may or may not heal depending on the underlying nature of the disease, extent of deformity, and general health of the individual.

Articular cartilage has no blood supply. When damaged, it is either replaced by fibrocartilage, which is not as smooth, or not replaced at all. Since articular cartilage also has no nerve supply, pain does not occur unless the underlying (subchondral) bone or synovial tissue is involved. Articular cartilage injuries are relatively permanent, although function can be preserved with replacement by fibrocartilage. Articular cartilage injuries are usually accompanied by subtle joint instability and synovial (joint capsule) inflammation, a clinical syndrome known as arthritis. Significant damage to the articular cartilage, subchondral bone, and synovium may require surgical replacement with an artificial joint.

Connective Tissue, Epithelium, and Endothelium

Normal Morphology and Physiology

Connective tissue consists of *collagen* and *elastin*. It attaches body structures, such as organs, bones, and muscles, to one another. A higher proportion of collagen indicates relatively greater tensile strength but less flexibility, whereas the opposite is true for a higher proportion of elastin. Connective tissue, although highly vascular and innervated, usually only has a few living cells interspersed in the tissue.

Epithelium lines the interior and exterior surfaces of the body, including the skin, gastrointestinal tract, and pulmonary system. Epithelium provides a barrier to the external environment. *Endothelium* lines the cardiovascular system, including the heart, arteries, veins, and lymphatic system. Endothelium regulates the exchange of substances, including nutrients, metabolic waste products, gases, infectious microorganisms, and toxins, between the blood and other organs. Both epithelium and endothelium have several specialized cell subtypes and exist in various cell thicknesses throughout the body. The rate of replication for these cells is very high. Thus, relatively new cells are constantly being moved to the surface to replace older cells that may have been exposed to potentially toxic, infectious, or damaging substances.

Pathological Processes

Physical damage or infection causes cell damage in these tissues. Metabolic diseases are also relatively common in connective tissue (eg, rheumatoid arthritis, gout, vasculitis) and cause chronic inflammation, tissue destruction, and scarring. Epithelium and endothelium are prone to cancer and toxic damage due to their constant exposure to the environment (indirectly through the blood in the case of endothelium). Particularly troublesome with damaged epithelium or endothelium cells are changes in tissue permeability, resulting in either inappropriate substances entering the body or inhibition of appropriate substances being exchanged.

Response to Injury or Disease

Connective, epithelial, and endothelial tissues very closely follow the "typical" inflammatory and infectious responses previously outlined. Connective tissue heals with collagen only. Hence, any tissue with elastin as a primary component loses flexibility after injury and healing. This effect may also interfere with organ function. For instance, collagen scars in the abdomen following surgery can sometimes cause a stricture (or narrowing) of the intestinal passageway, thus restricting passage of food.

Collagen scar tissue usually provides the same tensile strength as the original connective tissue within 6 to 8 weeks, provided the optimal healing environment (nutrients and oxygen from the blood) is present and the tissue is protected from reinjury. Remodeling of the collagen tissue to arrange fiber alignment consistent with the original structure, however, may take 6 to 12 months. Since collagen aligns along lines of consistent tissue stretch, thus providing higher tensile strength, appropriate functional demands should be placed on the tissue through this period.

Injured epithelium and endothelium can be replaced with normal cells, provided the damage does not extend through all cell layers and the genetic mechanism is not affected. The healing process takes a few days to close the wound, a few weeks to return to full strength, and several months to remodel completely. Function of the resulting scar is dependent on the extent of the injury. A larger injury, resulting in a larger scar, will have a greater impairment of tissue function. If all cell layers are damaged, the tissue is replaced by nonfunctional collagen scar (metaplasia). If the DNA replication mechanism is affected, a cancerous lesion forms (dysplasia). Replacement of living cells with inflexible collagen not only leads to possible restrictions or obstructions, as noted above, but also causes the tissue to be nonpermeable, preventing normal cellular exchange. Cancerous changes can also cause obstructions and interfere with normal tissue function.

Table 2-2		
MUSCLE CELL TYPES, LOCATION, AND FUNCTION		
Type	*Body System*	*Function*
Striated	Musculoskeletal	Movement of the bones and body through space
Cardiac	Heart	Maintain blood flow to the body
Smooth	Vascular and gastrointestinal	Movement of blood and food through the respective systems

Muscle and Nerve

Normal Morphology and Physiology

Muscle tissue is comprised of one of three types of muscle cells: striated, cardiac, and smooth (Table 2-2). The principle function of muscle is contraction, which moves the skeleton, circulates the blood, or moves food through the bowels. Nerve cells transmit electrical signals that are initiated by external or internal stimuli. These signals control the movement, cognitive, and regulatory systems of the body. Nerve cells within the brain and associated structures are highly specialized, whereas the structure of nerve cells in the peripheral nervous system are similar to one another. All nerve cells contain a cell body, dendrites (projections that receive signals from other cells), and axons (projections that send signals to other cells). Chemical processes form the electrical impulses within (primarily through sodium ion exchanges) and between (via neurotransmitters) cells.

Pathological Processes

Skeletal muscle is most commonly affected by physical trauma (contusion or strain) or infection (eg, tetanus), although genetic and metabolic diseases also occur (eg, muscular dystrophy, myesthesia gravis). In contrast, cardiac and smooth muscle are more commonly affected by metabolic states (such as ischemia) and infection. Toxins can also affect the various types of muscle, nervous tissue, or the neuromuscular junction.

Nerve cells are easily damaged by physical trauma, toxins, infections, and metabolic imbalances. Many pathological processes directly or indirectly affect the nervous system. Thus, signs of nervous system impairment are often early indications of systemic disease. In addition, some diseases affect the biochemical mechanisms that propagate electrical impulses. In such instances, cell structure is maintained, although cell function is impaired.

Response to Injury or Disease

Muscle cell response to damage is similar to that of connective tissue. Damaged cells and tissue are replaced by collagen tissue rather than normal contractile muscle. Depending on severity and extent of injury, a large noncontractile scar within a muscle can be quite disabling. If a relatively small proportion of skeletal muscle tissue is damaged, however, resistance training of the remaining muscle tissue can compensate. If a significant proportion of the smooth muscle of internal organs or cardiac muscle is damaged, however, severe impair-

Table 2-3

EXAMPLES OF SPECIALIZED CELL TYPES, LOCATIONS, AND FUNCTIONS

Cell Type	Location	Function
Mucosa	Gastrointestinal	Absorb nutrients, secrete mucus for protection and enzymes for digestion
Acinar	Exocrine pancreas	Secrete digestive enzymes
Islet	Endocrine pancreas	Alpha cells secrete glucagon, beta cells secrete insulin
Hepatic	Liver	Secretes bile, stores carbohydrates, forms urea; metabolism of cholesterol, lipids, and many drugs and toxins
Renal	Kidney	Regulate fluid, form urine
Endocrine	Endocrine glands	Secrete regulatory specific hormones

ment or complete loss of function occurs in the associated organ. Irreversible damage to muscle of internal organs, particularly the heart, can be fatal.

Unfortunately, damage to the body of a nerve cell is permanent. A nerve cell can neither be replaced nor regenerated, resulting in permanent loss of the functions associated with that nerve cell. Damage to any portion of the nerve cell (dendrite, axon, or body) in the central nervous system (brain and spinal cord) is also permanent. If an axon is damaged in the peripheral nervous system, however, it can regenerate provided the myelin (a lipoprotein) sheath surrounding the axon is preserved and aligned. The axon first degenerates distal to the point of injury and then regenerates inside the myelin sheath at a rate of approximately .25 inch per month.

Specialized Cells and Tissues

Normal Morphology and Physiology

Cells of the blood, gastrointestinal system, liver, kidneys, and endocrine glands are highly specialized and perform specific tasks (Table 2-3). Most of the functions are integral to larger systems or the overall homeostatic mechanism. Thus, abnormal function in one of the systems usually (eventually) affects one or more of the other systems. Pathology in these organs often produces the systemic signs reviewed in Table 1-7, which reflects the functional interaction of these systems.

Pathological Processes

Pathology of gastrointestinal, liver, or kidney cells can be caused by infection, metabolic or genetic changes, or toxicity. Direct physical trauma, which is perhaps most common in young people and athletes, can disrupt tissues and interfere with organ function. Blood cells can also be affected by infection, metabolic changes, or toxicity, and can be indirectly affected by trauma to other tissues. Substantial tissue trauma may cause a loss of large amounts of blood from the vascular system, called *hemorrhage*. Hemorrhage has serious and potentially fatal consequences as organs become progressively deprived of bloodborne nutrients and oxygen, a process known as *shock* (see Chapter Three). The signs of shock reflect the homeostatic effort to maintain blood volume in the internal organs, including pallor and cool (clammy) skin from peripheral vasoconstriction, hypotension (low blood pressure) from low blood volume within the vascular system, and tachycardia (increased heart rate) in an effort to maintain blood flow to the organs of the body. Shock can also be caused by a response to heart failure (decreasing systemic blood flow) or widespread peripheral vasodilatation (in response to autonomic nervous system action, systemic infection, or anaphylaxis).

Endocrine glands are rarely affected by trauma, but physical damage may occur with major injuries and diseases in surrounding organs. More commonly, genetic factors induce abnormal function or tumor development. Environmental factors also potentially affect endocrine function through toxicity. Tumors in the endocrine glands can either reduce or increase secretion of specific hormones, thus upsetting metabolic homeostasis. In addition, since hormones affect multiple organs, signs and symptoms are produced in several systems.

Response to Injury or Disease

The tissues of the gastrointestinal organs, liver, and kidneys are highly vascularized and display a typical inflammatory response in reaction to cellular damage. This inflammation produces clinical signs specific to the functions of the affected organ or organs (see Chapters Five and Six). These cells have a limited ability to regenerate, but if chronic cell damage and inflammation persists, the damage becomes permanent and cells are replaced by fibrous tissue. With repeated, prolonged, or severe damage, the organs can no longer function properly and may restrict blood flow to surrounding healthy cells, thus propagating cell damage. Examples of this type of pathology include cirrhosis of the liver, chronic renal failure, and inflammatory bowel disease.

Blood Cells

The presence of infection (septicemia) or a toxin in the blood causes a vigorous inflammatory response throughout the body. The high fever produced in such a condition can destroy other tissues, posing a serious threat to homeostasis and life. The blood can also be affected by genetic diseases, including sickle cell anemia (misshapen red blood cells) and leukemia (proliferation of immature blood cells). These diseases also cause a mild or moderate general inflammatory response.

SUMMARY

Pathophysiology refers to the biological process of disease. The mechanism called homeostasis responds to the changing internal and external environment to maintain chemical, fluid, and energy balances in the body. Many pathological processes upset this equilibrium. The basic unit of the body is the cell. Virtually all pathological processes can be expressed in terms of their effect on individual cells. Cells can be damaged by physical, infective, metabolic, genetic, or environmental factors, causing them to either adapt or die. When enough cells die, tissue, organ, and system functions are affected. Inflammation and infection are general responses to cell damage. Each cell and tissue type also produces specific responses to the various types of damage. Signs and symptoms are the manifestations of the general and specific responses to cell damage.

REFERENCES

1. Gould BE. *Introduction to Pathophysiology. Pathophysiology for the Health-Related Professions.* Philadelphia, Pa: WB Saunders Company; 1997:3-8.

2. Majno G, ed. *Cells, Tissues, and Disease: Principles of General Pathology.* Cambridge, Mass: Blackwell Science Inc; 1996.

3. Sell S, ed. *Immunology, Immunopathology & Immunity,* 5th ed. Stamford, Conn: Appleton & Lange; 1996.

4. Shaw M, Roy CM, Bartelmo JM, Hendler C, et al, eds. *Pathophysiology Made Incredibly Easy.* Springhouse, Pa: Springhouse Corporation; 1998.

5. Underwood JCE, ed. *General and Systematic Pathology.* 2nd ed. New York: Churchill Livingstone; 1996.

6. Ganong WF. *Review of Medical Physiology.* 15th ed. Norwalk, Conn: Appleton & Lange; 1991.

Chapter Three

Cardiovascular and Hematological Systems

PURPOSES

- Describe basic cardiovascular structures and their functions.
- Review pathophysiological mechanisms of the cardiovascular system.
- Describe the response of the cardiovascular system to exercise.
- Discuss medical history results that are relevant to cardiovascular pathology.
- Identify signs and symptoms of cardiac pathology.
- Identify signs and symptoms of vascular pathology.
- Identify signs and symptoms of pathology of the blood.
- Perform physical examination tasks relevant to the cardiovascular system.
- Discuss, compare, and contrast selected pathological conditions of the cardiovascular system.

INTRODUCTION

The occurrence of cardiovascular disease has declined in the United States over the past 20 years, but heart disease and stroke remain among the leading causes of death.[1] Through ambitious public health education, many cardiovascular risk factors such as smoking, high blood pressure, high blood cholesterol, and diabetes have been significantly reduced in the population. Despite the protective effects of exercise, however, cardiovascular events cause most "on the field" sudden deaths among athletes.[2-4] One of the primary purposes of a preparticipation physical examination is to detect and counsel athletes who may be at risk for a cardiac incident.[4,5]

The American College of Sports Medicine (ACSM) and the American Heart Association (AHA) recommend that all persons who exercise regularly should be routinely evaluated for signs of potential cardiovascular disease.[6] This is particularly important for physically active people over the age of 35 years, for whom coronary artery disease is the leading cause of exercise-associated death.[2,3,5-8] Athletic trainers should therefore be able to detect signs and symptoms of cardiovascular pathology and be prepared to respond in a cardiac emergency.

REVIEW OF PHYSIOLOGY AND PATHOGENESIS

The cardiovascular system consists of the heart and blood vessels, including arteries, veins, and lymph vessels. Blood, the principal organ of the hematological system, is functionally related to the cardiovascular system and will also be discussed in this chapter. The heart (Figure 3-1), a four-chambered organ made of special muscle called myocardium, pumps blood to every organ of the body. Muscular septa, or walls, separate the left and right atria in the superior part of the heart and separate the left and right ventricles, which lie inferior to the respective atrium. A sac of connective tissue, called the endocardium, encloses the entire heart. Tissue called pericardium attaches the endocardium (and the heart) to the thorax. Potential pathology affecting the myocardium includes heart failure, cardiomyopathy, congenital defects, trauma, and ischemia (a loss of blood supply). The endocardium and pericardium are subject to infection and edema.

Arteries, veins, and lymphatics circulate the various body fluids (Figure 3-2). All have three layers: an inner layer (tunica intima) of endothelium, a middle layer (tunica media) of elastic fibers and smooth muscle, and an outer layer (tunica adventitia) of connective tissue. The relative thickness of these layers, as well as the proportion of elastic fibers or smooth muscle, depends on the vessel type and location in the body.

Arteries, which carry oxygenated blood from the heart, are classified as either muscular or elastic. Arteries with a large portion of muscle can regulate blood flow to specific organs. The major arteries of the trunk, however, are elastic to accommodate pressure suddenly rising during heart contraction. This elasticity also assists blood flow during heart relaxation.

Veins, which return blood to the heart, have very little muscle. Blood flow toward the heart is supported by skeletal muscle contraction, which creates pressure in veins. Lower pressure in the thorax (during inspiration) also draws blood toward the heart. In addition, venous valves prevent back flow of blood.

The lymphatic system drains and filters body fluids (lymph), absorbs and transports fat, and participates in the immune response. Lymph nodes are small expansions within the lymph vessels. All lymph travels through at least one node before entering the bloodstream

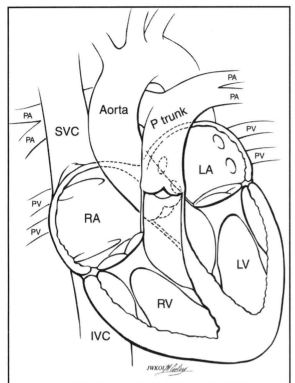

Figure 3-1. Structure of the heart.

Key: LA = left atrium; RA = right atrium; LV = left ventricle; RV = right ventricle; SVE = superior vena cava; IVC = inferior vena cava; P trunk = pulmonary trunk

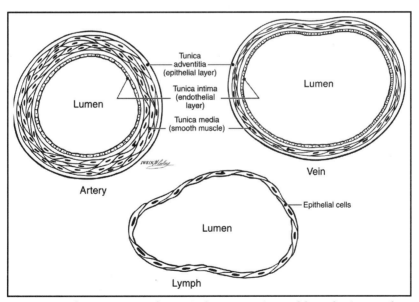

Figure 3-2. Cross-section of a typical artery, vein, and lymphatic vessel.

Figure 3-3. Cardiac conduction system.

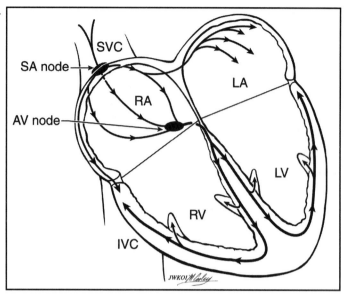

just proximal to the superior vena cava. Lymph flow occurs by the same mechanisms as venous flow.

Heart muscle requires oxygen and other nutrients, as do all living tissues. The coronary arteries branch immediately from the base of the aorta to supply the entire myocardium. The left coronary artery is larger than the right and thus supplies a greater proportion of the heart. Congenital deformities of the coronary arteries pose a threat during vigorous exercise. Pathology affecting the rest of the vascular system includes obstructive diseases, peripheral vascular disease, abnormal vasomotor responses, congenital malformations, and aneurysms.

The heartbeat begins as an electrical discharge, which causes a wave of muscular contraction. First, the sinoatrial (SA) node depolarizes (electrically discharges) and spreads electricity through pathways in the atria, causing them to contract. When depolarization reaches the atrioventricular (AV) node, it is transmitted into the ventricular walls, as seen in Figure 3-3. The contraction of the ventricles pumps blood into the aorta and pulmonary arteries. Pathology affecting this conduction system changes the rhythm, pattern, or effectiveness of contraction. An electrocardiogram (ECG) detects electric activity of the heart and can identify these conditions.

The heart's mechanical action circulates blood to every cell in the body. *Diastole* refers to the period when the atria and ventricles are both relaxed, as opposed to *systole*, the contraction phase. During diastole, blood flows into the atria and through to the ventricles. At least 70% of ventricular filling occurs during this phase.

Atrial contraction (atrial systole) precedes ventricular contraction (ventricular systole). Atrial contraction begins after SA node depolarization. The mitral and tricuspid valves open as atrial pressure (Figure 3-4a) pushes blood into the ventricles. During ventricular contraction, the mitral and tricuspid valves close off the atria. The aortic and pulmonary valves open and blood flows into the respective vessels (Figure 3-4b). As the ventricles relax, the aortic and pulmonary valves close, and the next cardiac contraction begins. The amount of blood pumped into the aorta during a single ventricular contraction is *stroke volume*. Stroke vol-

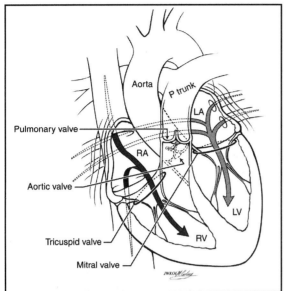

Figure 3-4a. Schematic of heart valves.

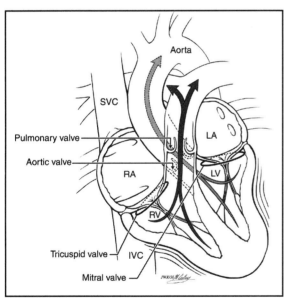

Figure 3-4b. Schematic of heart valves.

ume multiplied by heart rate (beats per minute) yields cardiac output, the volume of blood pumped per minute.

Blood circulates through the entire body. Table 3-1 lists the basic blood cells and their functions. Most blood cells form in the red bone marrow of long and flat bones. Many diseases and pathological states affect blood cells. Blood pressure (BP) maintains blood flow and perfusion of the head, internal organs, and muscles. With low blood pressure, the brain suffers from lack of oxygen. Conversely, high blood pressure eventually damages capillaries in many parts of the body. Table 3-2 summarizes some basic factors and mechanisms affecting blood pressure.

Table 3-1

BLOOD CELLS AND THEIR FUNCTIONS

Cell Type	Function
Red blood cells (erythrocytes)	Carry oxygen
White blood cells (lymphocytes)	Phagocytosis, immediate immune system response
Platelets (thrombocytes)	Clotting

Table 3-2

BASIC FACTORS AFFECTING BLOOD PRESSURE

Factor	Effect on BP	Mechanism
Decreased blood volume	Decrease	Inadequate fluid within the vascular system to maintain pressure
Widespread vasodilation	Decrease	Systemic capacity exceeds fluid volume
Increased extracellular fluid	Increase	Higher BP needed to diffuse nutrients against the increased pressure gradient in the capillaries
Renal failure	Increase	Higher BP needed to diffuse fluids against the increased pressure gradient in the kidney capillaries

Responses and Adaptations to Exercise

Exercising muscles require much more oxygen than they do at rest. Thus, heart rate and respiration rate both increase significantly once exercise begins, which increases demand on the heart. Regular aerobic exercise increases left ventricular mass and volume. This adaptation allows increased demands on the heart, greater venous return, and increased oxygen delivery to the body.[9] Resistance exercise also increases the muscle mass of the left ventricle to adapt to increased resistance to blood flow. Oxygen demand, however, does not increase with resistance training, so the volume of the left ventricle does not change significantly.[9]

Preparticipation Screening

Appropriate preparticipation screening identifies persons who may be at risk for a cardiac event.[6] This may be done with simple questionnaires, such as the Physical Activity Readiness Questionnaire or the Health/Fitness Facility Preparticipation Screening Questionnaire.[6]

Athletes of high school or college age should be examined by a physician at least every other year before participation, including a medical history, auscultation of the heart and lungs, and resting blood pressure.[5] The history should include questions about exertional chest pain, fainting (syncope), light-headedness, dizziness, and family history of sudden or cardiac-related death. Positive responses to these questions may identify up to 50% of at-risk athletes, particularly if these symptoms interrupt a workout.[3,7]

The full report of the 26th Bethesda Conference, which provides medical recommendations for athletic eligibility for persons with cardiac conditions, is available through the American College of Cardiology, Heart House, 9111 Old Georgetown Rd, Bethesda, MD 20814-1699. Summaries of this report were published in a 1994 special issue of *Medicine and Science in Sports and Exercise.*[8,10-14]

SIGNS AND SYMPTOMS

Chest Pain

Chest pain is the principal symptom of cardiac pathology. This pain occurs over the left chest and radiates to the left neck, shoulder, or arm. It may be described as pressure that worsens with physical exertion. Autonomic responses such as diaphoresis or pallor may also appear.

Dyspnea

Shortness of breath occurs with decreased cardiac output, as oxygen available to the body decreases. Dyspnea nearly always improves with rest and worsens with activity. Cardiac-related dyspnea is unaffected by posture, whereas sitting relieves dyspnea from pulmonary disorders.

Fatigue

As when cardiac output decreases, the cells of the body slowly adapt by decreasing metabolism (the utilization of energy and oxygen). The effect is a reduction in the body's capability to perform work. The overall effect is called *fatigue.*

Palpitations

Palpitations describe the sensation of "skipped beats" or of the heart "fluttering" uncomfortably. Disturbance of the electrical activity of the heart (arrhythmia) causes palpitations. Palpitations accompanied by angina, dyspnea, fatigue, or light-headedness suggest a cardiac condition.

Syncope

Syncope, or fainting, is a complete loss of consciousness and loss of postural tone produced by a sudden reduction in the brain's blood supply. There are three main causes of syncope. The first is sudden peripheral vasodilatation, known as orthostatic syncope. The rapid perfusion of the extremities decreases blood supply to the brain, causing loss of consciousness. A second cause is increased intracranial pressure from intracranial bleeding, which prevents adequate blood flow to the cerebrum. The third cause is an acute reduction in cardiac output (heart failure). Spontaneous syncope indicates serious arrhythmia or heart disease and requires emergency medical care.

Other medical conditions, such as seizures, metabolic disorders, poisoning, and neurological disorders, can cause a change in level of consciousness. These syndromes, however, are not considered true syncope since either the loss of consciousness or the loss of postural tone is not complete.

Claudication

Claudication, literally meaning a state of impaired gait, occurs when blood flow in lower limb arteries is blocked. Consequently, oxygen does not reach the muscles in sufficient quantity. Claudication produces cramping, aching, and unusual limb fatigue.

Skin and Nail Temperature, Color, and Appearance

Vasomotor disorders can cause the skin to become notably cool (clammy) or hot, or to change colors, ranging from very pale to bright red to blue or purple. Persons in shock or experiencing a severe cardiac event often have pale and clammy skin. Various chronic cardiovascular disorders cause ulcers or lesions on the skin and "clubbing" (rounding) of the fingertips and nails (Figure 3-5).

Paresthesia

Although usually associated with neurologic pathology, *paresthesia* (abnormal sensation) can result from obstruction of blood flow to an extremity.

Edema

Edema, the presence of fluid in interstitial spaces, occurs with chronic cardiac conditions or obstruction of veins or lymph vessels. In both situations, excess fluid in the blood moves from the vessels into the surrounding tissues. Cardiac failure causes generalized edema, whereas vascular conditions cause edema distal to the obstruction.

PAIN PATTERNS

Cardiac

The heart produces pain in spinal levels C3 through T4, anywhere from the neck and throat to the medial side of the left arm. Most often, a "crushing" or pressure sensation begins in the chest and radiates to the left arm (Figure 3-6).

Vascular

Vascular pain, described as tearing, sharp, or throbbing, occurs in the region of the affected vessel. Secondary symptoms appear when tissues supplied by the pathological vessel are

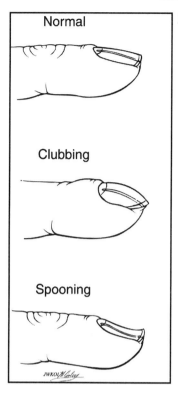

Normal

Clubbing

Spooning

Figure 3-5. Clubbing and spooning of the fingernails.

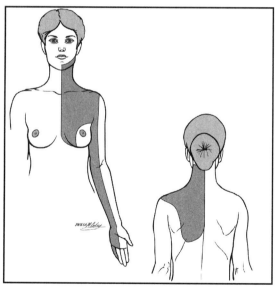

Figure 3-6. Cardiac pain pattern.

affected. These symptoms depend on the affected tissue or organ system. Muscles cramp, weaken, or fatigue, nerves experience paresthesia, and internal organs cease or alter their respective functions.

MEDICAL HISTORY AND PHYSICAL EXAMINATION

Family and Personal History

A history of sudden cardiac death under age 40 in the immediate family may indicate an underlying cardiac abnormality.[5] A *personal history* of physical inactivity, smoking, hypertension, high blood lipids, obesity, diabetes, Marfan's syndrome, or connective tissue disorders increases the probability of developing cardiovascular pathology.[1,3,6] Among studies of sudden death among athletes, many reported a positive family history and about 20% reported signs or symptoms, such as exertional angina, dyspnea, syncope, unusual fatigue, palpitations, a known heart murmur, or increased blood pressure, before their fatal event.[2-5,7,15]

Symptoms

Pain of cardiac origin is either acute (sudden and severe) and constant or subacute (insidious and moderate) and recurrent. Cardiac pain is described as a crushing pressure that starts in the chest. Chest pain associated with exertion also indicates cardiac pathology.[16,17] Pain associated with pathology of the pericardium becomes worse in supine and improves when sitting.[16]

Chest pain radiating into the arm, throat, jaw, or back that lasts between 2 to 10 minutes (angina) is a hallmark of ischemic cardiac pathology.[18] Up to 30% of people with sudden angina at rest have a myocardial infarction (heart attack) within 3 months. Anyone reporting unexplained syncope, palpitations, or dyspnea, particularly with chest pain or during exertion, may have cardiovascular pathology and needs referral for medical examination.[5,18]

Symptoms of vascular pathology include cramping, heaviness, weakness, swelling, pulsing or fatigue, or cold or cyanotic extremities. These symptoms worsen with exertion and are relieved by rest.[19-23]

Inspection

Certain physical characteristics are associated with cardiovascular conditions. For instance, 80% to 90% of people with Marfan's syndrome develop deformities in the aorta, which could lead to rupture and death (Table 3-3).[9,11,24,25] In addition, the aortic and mitral valves may be affected, producing "clicks" upon auscultation.[24,25] Any two physical signs of Marfan's syndrome warrants referral for medical cardiac screening.[25]

A lack of the normal thoracic kyphosis, or a deformed or displaced sternum, may also indicate congenital heart abnormalities.[26] Any notable deformity of the chest wall in a child should be examined by a physician.

Auscultation

Auscultation involves using a stethoscope to listen to internal body sounds. Cardiac auscultation, described in Lab Activity 2 (page 233),[2-4,15,16,26,27] can detect "noises" other than

---

Table 3-3

SIGNS OF MARFAN'S SYNDROME

- Tall, thin body type
- Arm span longer than height
- Disproportionately long legs
- Thoracic spine kyphosis
- Sternum deformity (pectus carnitum, pectus excavatum)
- Hyperlaxity in joints
- Visual problems

---

the normal, rhythmic "lub-dub" of the heart valves. The first sound corresponds to the closing of the mitral and tricuspid valves as ventricular systole begins. The second sound corresponds to the aortic and pulmonary valves closing at the end of ventricular systole. Abnormal cardiac sounds include "extra" heart sounds, muffled heart sounds, rubbing, or hissing caused by valve deformities and murmurs.

The major vessels, such as the abdominal aorta, brachial arteries, and femoral arteries, can also be auscultated. Normally, the sound of the heartbeat may be faintly detectable, accompanied by the cyclic rushing sound of blood flow. Abnormal vascular sounds, called *bruits*, include loud clicks, pounding, or continuous rushing sounds. Increased turbulence in arteries that have been pathologically narrowed (atherosclerosis) or deformed (aneurysm) produce bruits.

Heart Rate

Heart rate, the number of heart beats per minute (bpm), can be palpated over the heart apex, at pulse-pressure sites (brachial, femoral, radial, dorsal pedis, etc), or the carotid artery. When assessing heart rate, the rate, rhythm (regular versus irregular), and character (strong versus weak) should be reported (eg, "120 bpm, regular and weak").

Normal heart rate ranges between 70 and 100 bpm. A slow resting heart rate is called *bradycardia* and a high resting heart rate is termed *tachycardia*. Normal cardiac rhythm should be regular and strong. Weak or irregular (skipping beats) pulse is an indicator of potential cardiac emergency. Resting bradycardia (< 60 bpm) occurs among trained athletes and is not generally a concern.[2,3] Likewise, rapid heart rate is normal during exercise but should return to normal range within a few minutes after stopping exercise. A heart rate at rest in excess of 100 beats per minute should be considered abnormal and requires physician referral.[18]

Respiration Rate

The respiration rate is normally 10 to 15 breaths per minute and can be easily evaluated while assessing heart rate or blood pressure. Respiration at rest should be regular, moderate in depth, and require little effort. Forced or difficult respiration, obvious dyspnea, or rapid, shallow breaths are abnormal. Chapter Four discusses assessment of respiration and pulmonary function.

Figure 3-7. Location of pulse sites.

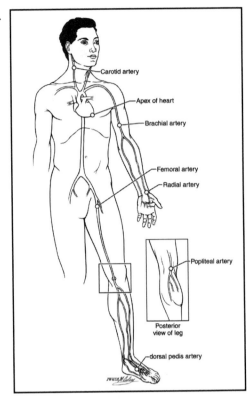

Blood Pressure

Blood pressure (BP) measures the pressure inside the arteries during systole and diastole. BP is usually measured at the brachial artery with an instrument called a sphygmomanometer as described in Lab Activity 3 (page 234).[3,4,15,18]

Normally, systolic BP ranges from 100 to 140 mmHg and diastolic BP ranges from 70 to 90 mmHg. BP equal to or greater than 140/90 on consecutive days indicates hypertension (high blood pressure) and needs further medical assessment.[18] Drastic differences in resting BP (more than 15 mmHg) between lying, sitting, and standing postures suggests neurological or cardiovascular pathology.

Palpation

Arterial pulses can be palpated where major arteries are close to the skin (Figure 3-7). Pulses may be absent or diminished in vascular occlusion syndromes. Aneurysms may be palpated as a "throbbing mass" on the affected artery. A palpable abdominal pulse wider than the normal aortic pulsation (2 inches to either side of the midline) may indicate aortic aneurysm. Palpable, swollen, tender, or hard lymphatic vessels or lymph nodes (lymphadenitis) are never normal, but indicate infection, trauma, or occlusion.

PATHOLOGY AND PATHOGENESIS

Sudden (Cardiac) Death

The incidence of exercise-induced death is relatively small, ranging from 1 in 50,000 to 200,000 in males, and 1 in 200,000 to 769,000 in females of high school or collegiate age.[4,7,9,15,28] Nontraumatic sudden cardiac death presents symptoms within 1 hour of sport activity. Congenital coronary artery anomalies, hypertrophic cardiomyopathy, electrical and conduction abnormalities, or acquired myocarditis are the most common causes of sudden death in athletes.[1-3,5-9,15,28] Some contributing risk factors include the physiological stress of exercise, electrolyte imbalances (a consequence of dehydration), high body temperature (from exercise in extreme heat and humidity), and sudden cessation of intense activity (causing vasodilatation and falling BP, similar to shock).[3,5,9,15]

Other causes of sudden cardiac death include aortic rupture (associated Marfan's syndrome), aortic stenosis, congenital cerebrovascular deformities, pulmonary disease, peripheral embolism, and drug abuse.[2-4,7,9,15] Blunt trauma to the chest can induce a severe ventricular arrhythmia called *commotio cordis*, particularly if an underlying structural abnormality exists.[3] Commotio cordis has virtually no possibility of resuscitation.[9]

Disorders of the Myocardium and Coronary Arteries

Heart Failure

When cardiac output decreases because of an insufficient heart pump mechanism, the resulting condition is called heart failure. Several types of heart failure are identified by the side of the heart that is affected (left or right) and whether the failure is acute or chronic. Acute heart failure is immediately life threatening, whereas patients with chronic heart failure display gradual but progressive systemic failures. Table 3-4 summarizes the respective effects of these conditions. *Cor pulmonale* is the term used for right heart failure as a consequence of pulmonary disease.[29] Signs and symptoms of cor pulmonale are similar to chronic right heart failure accompanied by signs of pulmonary disease (see Chapter Four).

Myocardial Ischemia

An imbalance between myocardial oxygen demand and coronary artery oxygen supply causes angina. Any condition that limits myocardial blood supply can cause this effect. For example, abnormal formation of the coronary arteries can cause angina as well as dyspnea and syncope during exercise.[2,3,5,9,15]

Coronary artery disease (CAD), including arteriosclerosis, comprises the majority of cardiac deaths among physically active persons over 35 years of age.[4,9] If CAD obstructs the coronary arteries, the associated myocardium becomes ischemic and necrotic, a condition called myocardial infarction (MI). A significant proportion of MIs occur during moderate to heavy activity, such as manual labor or athletics.[7]

Ischemic disorders affecting the myocardium usually exhibit typical cardiac signs and symptoms, including angina, unusual fatigue, dizziness, or syncope.[2-4,9] In an acute cardiac emergency, vital signs (heart rate, respiration rate, BP) change rapidly. A person with these signs should be withdrawn from participation and referred for emergency medical care.

Table 3-4

TYPES OF HEART FAILURE, CONSEQUENCES, AND SIGNS

Location	Consequences	Signs
Acute left	Usually associated with MI Failure to deliver blood to the body Pulmonary edema	Dyspnea, pulmonary edema, pink frothy sputum, cyanosis, and hypotension
Chronic left	Failure to deliver blood to the body Pulmonary edema	Dyspnea with exertion and during sleep, unusual fatigue, tachycardia, cool skin, cyanosis, pulmonary edema
Acute right	Usually with pulmonary embolism Failure to deliver blood to the lungs Systemic edema	Cool skin, hypotension, cyanosis
Chronic right	Failure to deliver blood to the lungs Systemic edema	Dyspnea, fatigue, abdominal discomfort, decreased appetite, and peripheral edema

Hypertrophic Cardiomyopathy

Three types of cardiac hypertrophy, or enlargement of the heart (Figure 3-8), are recognized: general cardiac hypertrophy (both ventricles), left ventricular hypertrophy, and right ventricular hypertrophy. General cardiac hypertrophy in athletes is most commonly a normal adaptation to chronic aerobic exercise.[28] In pathological conditions (eg, hypertrophic cardiomyopathy), however, abnormal myocardial fibers form asymmetrical (eg, left or right) hypertrophy, causing ventricular obstruction and arrhythmia. An estimated 1 in 500 young adults display signs of potential hypertrophic cardiomyopathy.[2-5,7,15]

Eventually, hypertrophic cardiomyopathy leads to congestive heart failure, ischemic myocardial damage, or fatal arrhythmia.[1] Most people with these conditions have a family history of sudden death under age 50, or a personal history of unexplained episodes of syncope, angina, or dyspnea.[3,5,28] A murmur that increases with Valsalva's maneuver (see Lab Activity 2) is sometimes auscultated at the lower left sternal border, medial to the apex of the heart.[9,28,30] Definitive diagnosis is achieved through echocardiography.[2,4,28]

Hypertrophic cardiomyopathy is managed through medications, activity restriction, and surgery in certain cases.[31] Risk of arrhythmia increases with increased cardiac demand. Thus, the 26th Bethesda Conference recommends that an athlete with pathological cardiac hypertrophy withdraw from intense sport. Many athletes, however, ignore this precaution and choose to risk a fatal cardiac event.[13,15]

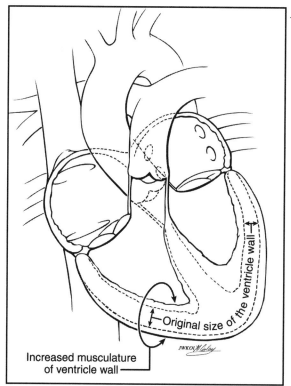

Figure 3-8. Cardiac hypertrophy.

Increased musculature of ventricle wall

Original size of the ventricle wall

Valve Disorders

Any of the valves of the heart (mitral, aortic, tricuspid, pulmonary) can be affected by congenital deformities or acquired disease. Two such disorders are stenosis (narrowing) that restricts blood flow through the valve (Figure 3-9) or structural malformations (eg, prolapse) that allow back flow of blood through the valve. Valve disorders cause murmurs on auscultation, the sound turbulent blood flow produces through the deformed valve. Heart valve disorders often occur with other cardiac or systemic diseases.

Generally, athletes with valve disorders who have normal heart rate and rhythm, normal heart size, and normal cardiac function are not excluded from participating in sports.[10] Those cases with more severe valve deformities that cause electrical (arrythmia) or structural changes (hypertrophy), or affect heart function, are judged based on severity of the disorders.[10]

Mitral valve prolapse (MVP), which is the most common valve disorder, is caused by deformed mitral valve leaflets that bulge back into the aorta during ventricular systole, thus allowing back flow of blood (Figure 3-9). Persons with MVP but without syncope, family history of sudden death, arrhythmia, substantial back flow, or previous cardiac-related events can participate in sports without restriction.[13]

Cardiac Conduction Disorders

Benign atrial arrhythmia occurs in some highly fit individuals as a result of exercise-induced bradycardia.[3] Pathological arrhythmia, however, is produced by abnormal or

Figure 3-9. Common valvular disorders.

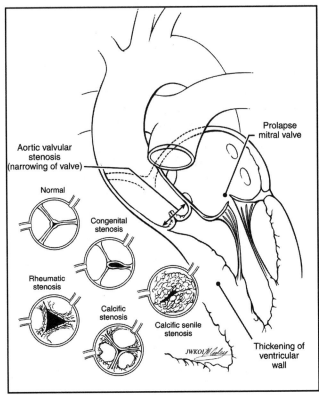

blocked conduction pathways, leading to ventricular fibrillation and acute heart failure.[5,32] Dangerous arrhythmias are diagnosed by ECG.

Most people with a significant arrhythmia will have exertional palpitations or syncope.[5,32] Syncope during exercise is highly suggestive of significant cardiac arrhythmia.[14] Athletes with symptomatic ventricular arrhythmia should be excluded from competition for at least 6 months and cleared by ECG before returning.[32] Qualification for sports depends on the type and severity of the arrhythmia and following established guidelines.[14]

Arrhythmogenic Right Ventricular Dysplasia

Arrhythmogenic right ventricular dysplasia (ARVD) is fatty infiltration (penetration) and fibrosis of the right ventricle.[5,9] ARVD has a genetic component and produces ventricular tachycardia or life-threatening ventricular arrhythmia.[5,9] Persons with ARVD may have a history of cardiac signs and symptoms upon exertion, often detectable during preparticipation examination.[9]

Hypertension

Hypertension (HTN) is defined as resting blood pressure (BP) greater than 140/90 on three consecutive occasions.[12,33] Mild hypertension is diastolic BP of 90 to 104 mmHg (or systolic 140 to 159 mmHg), moderate hypertension is diastolic BP between 105 and 114 mmHg (systolic 160 to 179 mmHg), and severe hypertension is diastolic BP over 115 mmHg (systolic over 180 mmHg).[26,29,33] Primary (essential) arterial HTN often has unknown pathogenesis, but genetic and environmental factors (eg, urban living, diet, obesity, chronic stress, smoking) contribute. Secondary HTN (resulting from another medical condition) is caused most often by renal, hormonal, or metabolic disorders.[29]

Many persons with HTN are asymptomatic, although some experience frequent occipital headaches and epistaxis (nosebleed). A headache occurs when diastolic pressure exceeds 120 mmHg. This headache is usually mild, present upon waking, and disappears with mild activity.[34] Extreme blood pressure responses during exercise (systolic pressure of 240 mmHg or greater) may be a sign of cardiovascular pathology.[35]

Long-term complications of HTN include heart disease, stroke, retinal damage, renal failure, and peripheral vascular disease.[29] Persons with mild to moderate HTN without associated organ damage or heart disease need not be restricted from participating in sports but should be reassessed at least every 2 to 4 months. Severe HTN requires avoidance of strenuous sports (eg, power lifting) until BP is controlled by lifestyle or medication and organ damage has been assessed.[12]

Acetylcholinesterase (ACE) inhibitors and calcium channel blockers that are often prescribed for HTN have no particular precautions relative to exercise restrictions. Patients on diuretics, however, need to be monitored for dehydration and those on beta blockers need close monitoring of heart rate, which is limited by the medication.[33] Regular aerobic exercise at 60% to 70% of maximum heart rate decreases resting BP, particularly for mild cases of HTN.[12,33]

Disorders of the Blood

Anemia

Anemia is medically defined as a hemoglobin level or red blood cell (RBC) volume (hematocrit) below the fifth percentile for age (ie, 95% of persons of a certain age have higher values).[36,37] Since hemoglobin in RBCs carries oxygen, anemia impairs oxygen transport and limits work capacity.[38] Anemia thereby affects physical and athletic performance.[37]

Primary risk factors for anemia include malnutrition and chronic disease. Other risk factors are disadvantaged socioeconomic status (leading to malnutrition), intense physical training (destruction of RBCs), prolonged use of analgesics (impaired RBC formation), positive family history, and increased menstrual flow (loss of RBCs).[37] Anemia produces pallor, swollen tongue, spooning (thin, concave) nails (see Figure 3-4), scaly lips with fissures at the edges, and impaired attention.[37] For competitive athletics, adolescent males should be screened for anemia at least once and females every 2 or 3 years.[37]

Dilutional anemia (also known as "sports anemia" or "pseudoanemia") is common among athletes. Since exercise increases blood plasma volume but does not affect RBC count, blood tests may indicate anemia (low RBC relative to blood volume). This type of anemia, however, is asymptomatic, not affected by iron supplementation, and does not affect performance (since total oxygen delivery is unaffected).[37,39]

Most studies indicate exercise neither causes nor exacerbates true anemia.[37] Chronic blood loss, most often through menstruation and increased by stress, intense exercise, and oral contraceptives, will lead to low blood iron, which may or may not occur with anemia. Mild iron deficiency alone will not affect physical performance.[37]

Sickle Cell Anemia

Sickle cell anemia (SCA) occurs as a recessive genetic trait, producing abnormally shaped RBCs that inhibit binding of oxygen.[40] The result, like all true anemias, is decreased oxygen delivery. Between 8% and 10% of African-Americans carry the genetic sickle cell trait, and about 1% develop sickle cell anemia.[40]

The relative risk of sudden death is 27 times higher among persons of African descent who carry the sickle cell trait than among persons of African descent without the trait, and 40 times higher than among other races.[9] Death can occur from emboli (sickled cells tend to clot easily) or sickle cell crises (producing organ infarction and shock). SCA is also a risk factor for acute exertional rhabdomyolysis (sudden catabolic destruction of skeletal muscle), which usually occurs during vigorous exercise in hot, humid weather.[9,41,42] In this condition, myoglobin (a muscle protein) and enzymes pour into the bloodstream. Acute renal failure, shock, and death may result.[42]

Hemophilia

Hemophilia is a genetic disorder that impairs blood-clotting ability. Several types of hemophilia are identified depending on the clotting components that are absent or ineffective in the blood. Some types lead to prolonged and severe blood loss and are therefore more dangerous for competitive athletes. The general recommendation for persons with severe forms of hemophilia is to avoid collision sports and some contact sports.[43] Furthermore, replacement therapy (replacement of blood-clotting components) is recommended to prevent severe hemorrhaging during sports participation. For persons with hemophilia, recovery from musculoskeletal injuries may take longer than expected.[43]

Vascular Disorders

Trauma

Repeated blunt trauma, particularly in the hand and fingers (eg, catching a baseball), damages capillaries and arterioles, producing ischemia distal to the injury.[22,44] Symptoms include hypersensitivity to cold, numbness, and asymmetric pallor of the affected region.[22,44] This condition is treated with rest, protective padding, avoidance of cold, and possibly vasodilatation medications.[44]

Occlusion Syndromes

Common sites of occlusion include the subclavian, axillary, popliteal, and femoral arteries.[20,23] Chronic arterial occlusion produces intermittent muscle cramps, diminished distal pulses, bruits upon auscultation, dystrophic skin and nails, ulcerations of the skin, and loss of hair in a distal area.[18] Acute arterial occlusion produces the "five P's": pain, pallor, pulselessness, paresthesia, and paralysis distal to the occlusion.

Thoracic Outlet Syndrome

Thoracic outlet syndrome occurs when the subclavian or axillary artery becomes occluded by the scalene muscles, between the clavicle and first rib, or under the pectoralis minor. History usually reveals repetitive strenuous overhead activity or postures with prolonged scapular protraction (eg, desk work). Symptoms include diffuse arm aching that increases with exertion, paresthesia that increases at night, easy fatigability of the limb, and intermittent swelling of the limb.[23] Clinical signs vary, but distal temperature changes, cyanosis, and positive clinical tests assessing distal (radial) pulses (such as Adson's test, military bracing, or repeated clenching of the fist with the hand overhead).[45,46]

Other occlusion syndromes can occur in athletes. Acute (following trauma) or chronic (intermittent with activity) compartment syndromes can occlude an artery in the fascial compartment. For example, compartment syndrome of the anterior compartment of the lower leg produces weak dorsiflexion, numbness of the first web space (between toes one and two), and weak or absent dorsal pedis pulse. Buerger's disease (thrombangitis obliterans), which is associated with tobacco use, causes segmental inflammation and occlusion of arterioles, resulting in signs of occlusion simultaneously in the distal upper and lower extremities, which subsides with cessation of tobacco use.[20]

Deep Vein Thrombosis and Pulmonary Embolism

Deep vein thrombosis (DVT) and pulmonary embolism (PE) can occur after casting or other immobilization. As blood pools in large veins, it forms a thrombus (mass of clotted blood cells). A thrombus moving through the circulation is called an embolus. Classic signs and symptoms of DVT in the lower extremity are severe calf tenderness, distended veins, distal edema, and pain with passive dorsiflexion (Homan's sign). Fewer than one-third of patients who have DVT, however, actually exhibit these symptoms.[47] To prevent DVT, walking or active range of motion exercises, particularly for the lower extremities, should be performed several times a day for persons who are immobilized or casted. If activity is not possible, treatments such as medication (anticoagulants) and intermittent compression may be used.[47] Once signs of DVT appear, however, activity may need to be restricted until medication decreases the thrombus.

PE occurs when the embolus travels to a lung, causing infarction and necrosis of lung tissue.[48] PE presents severe chest pain, dyspnea, cough or hemoptysis (bloody sputum with cough), diaphoresis, anxiety, and hyperpnea (over 20 breaths per minute). A PE affecting a large lung segment can produce syncope, shock, and death, and is therefore a medical emergency.[48-50] Most cases will slowly resolve if managed appropriately (ie, in a hospital).[48]

Aneurysm

An aneurysm is a weakness in the vessel wall, usually from arteriosclerosis or infection, causing a dilation of all layers of the vessel wall at that point (Figure 3-10).[20,51] Aneurysms produce pulsing pain, auscultated bruits, and asymmetrical distal pulses. They are susceptible to rupture, which causes severe internal hemorrhage, shock, and death if untreated. Common sites for aneurysms include the aorta (common in Marfan's syndrome, producing abdominal pain in addition to other aneurysm signs), the major vessels (iliac, subclavian), and cerebral arteries (producing neurological signs; see Chapter Eight).

A false aneurysm can occur after trauma in sports or other physical activity. The wall of the vessel is torn, causing hematoma that develops into a fibrous scar on the vessel (see Figure 3-10). The interior diameter (lumen) of the vessel, however, is unchanged, so blood flow is unaffected.[20] The bulging scar may compress nearby anatomical structures, such as nerves or other vessels. History includes a local traumatic injury that has not resolved as expected. A painful, pulsatile mass is often palpable, but distal pulses are normal.[19,20] Rest usually is all that is needed, although occasionally surgical excision is required.

Headaches

A migraine headache is a vascular event, causing intense throbbing pain, usually unilaterally, with associated symptoms of nausea, vomiting, photophobia (aversion to light), and phonophobia (aversion to sound).[34] Many who suffer migraines have a positive family history.

A cluster headache is an intense, gnawing pain that is deep and nonthrobbing in nature, usually unilateral around the eye. Lacrimation (tearing), rhinorrhea (runny nose) or nasal congestion, diaphoresis, unilateral pupillary constriction (miosis), ptosis (drooping eyelid), and psychomotor agitation may occur. An episode can last up to 45 minutes and may recur night-

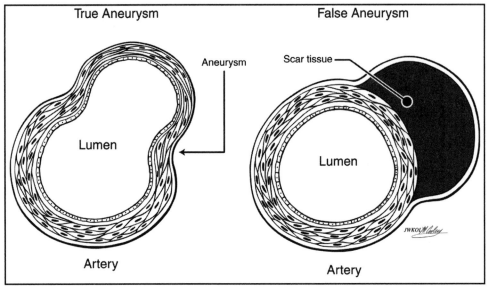

Figure 3-10. Aneurysm and false anuerysm.

ly.[34] Common exacerbating factors include psychoemotional stress and alcohol or tobacco use.

A toxic vascular headache presents diffuse, throbbing, severe pain over the entire crown.[34] Etiology includes infection (usually accompanied by fever), alcohol or caffeine abuse or withdrawal, hypoxia, hypoglycemia (low blood sugar), and metabolic disorders.[34]

Persons with vascular headaches are awake and alert, have no fever, and demonstrate a negative neurological examination (see Chapters One and Eight).[34] Treatment is rest in a quiet, dark room, and medication if chronic. If systemic signs and a severe headache occur simultaneously, emergency medical attention is required.

PEDIATRIC CONCERNS

Pediatric Chest Pain

Children rarely experience cardiac chest pain. Pediatric chest pain is usually a musculoskeletal condition or attributable to a specific event.[16] Asthma, depression, anxiety disorders, hyperventilation, autoimmune disease, anemia, school or family stress, or abuse may cause noncardiac chest pain. Children with a family history of heart disease who have chest pain, however, should be referred for medical examination.[16]

Congenital Heart Conditions

Most congenital heart problems are either septal wall defects or vascular anomalies. These disorders are often detected and surgically corrected during infancy, but more subtle cases are occasionally undetected.[5] Some children with heart conditions have a medical history of frequent illnesses, delayed growth, activity intolerance, malaise, and other chronic disease signs. Signs of potential cardiac pathology include fingernail clubbing, cyanosis, syncope, fatigue, dyspnea, and ausculated pericardial rub, murmurs, or clicks.[16]

Most congenital heart conditions are not adversely affected by exercise. Some exceptions are hypertrophic cardiomyopathy and congenital coronary artery anomalies (both very difficult to detect with routine screening examinations), cardiac complications of Marfan's syndrome, infective myocarditis, and major heart-vascular malformations.[11] Each child must be considered individually. Physical activity should be restricted only as necessary. In general, baseline and annual exercise testing with ECG and BP should be conducted to ascertain progression of disease as the child matures.[11] Again, the 26th Bethesda Conference guidelines can be consulted.[8,10-14]

SUMMARY

The cardiovascular system circulates blood, the principal organ of the hematological system. The hallmark of cardiac pathology is chest pain (angina) referring into the upper arm, anterior throat, face, jaw, and/or posterior chest wall. Other symptoms commonly associated with cardiac pathology include dyspnea, unusual fatigue, palpitations, and syncope. Symptoms of vascular pathology include changes in skin temperature, numbness, cramping, pain with activity, and limb fatigue during activity. The cardiovascular system can be examined using observation, auscultation, heart rate, palpation of pulses, and blood pressure. Pathology is possible in the myocardium (hypertrophic cardiomyopathy), coronary arteries (myocardial infarction), heart valves (murmurs), and cardiac conduction system (arrythmias) even among young, apparently healthy athletes. Anemia and hemophilia are hematological conditions that may be encountered among physically active persons. A careful preparticipation medical examination may identify persons at risk for a serious cardiovascular incident.

RESOURCES

Auscultation (Cardiac)

- Cardiac Auscultation site with audio of cardiac sounds. www.xs4all.nl/~medicine
- UCLA School of Medicine auscultation assistant site with audio of cardiac sounds. www.med.ucla.edu/wilkes/index.htm
- Virtual Stethoscope site with audio files for breath sounds (from McGill University). www.music.mcgill.ca/auscultation/auscultation.html

Cardiovascular

- American Heart Association (AHA). www.americanheart.org
- AHA's Heart and Stroke Guide. www.americanheart.org/Heart_and_Stroke_A_Z_Guide
- atlife.com cardiology site. www.atcardiology.com/cardiology

- Cardiac News on the Net updates of recent developments in cardiology. 207.158.219.110/cardiology.htm
- Vascular Web contains very basic information about the vascular system, including anatomy, physiology, and overview of diseases. www.rogers3.com/vascular
- *Yahoo* directories:

  dir.yahoo.com/Health/Diseases_and_Conditions/Heart_Diseases

  dir.yahoo.com/Health/Diseases_and_Conditions/Circulation_Diseases

  dir.yahoo.com/Health/Diseases_and_Conditions/Blood_Disorders

REFERENCES

1. National Institutes of Health Consensus Development Panel on Physical Activity and Cardiovascular Health. Physical activity and cardiovascular health. *JAMA.* 1996;276(3):241-246.

2. O'Connor FG, Kugler JP, Oriscello RG. Sudden death in young athletes: screening for the needle in a haystack. *Am Fam Physician.* 1998;57(11):2763-2770.

3. Franklin BA, Fletcher GF, Gordon NF, et al. Cardiovascular evaluation of the athlete: issues regarding performance, screening, and sudden cardiac death. *Sports Med.* 1997;24(2):97-119.

4. Maron BJ. Risk profiles and cardiovascular preparticipation screening of competitive athletes. *Cardiol Clin.* 1997;15(3):473-483.

5. Basilica FC. Cardiovascular disease in athletes. *Am J Sports Med.* 1999;27(1):108-121.

6. American College of Sports Medicine and American Heart Association. Recommendations for cardiovascular screening, staffing, and emergency policies at health/fitness facilities. *Med Sci Sports Exerc.* 1998;30(6):1009-1018.

7. Thompson PD. The cardiovascular complications of vigorous physical activity. *Arch Int Med.* 1996;156:2297-2302.

8. Thompson PD, Clock FJ, Leaven BD, et al. 26th Bethesda Conference: recommendations for determining eligibility for competition in athletes with cardiovascular abnormalities, task force 5: coronary artery disease. *Med Sci Sports Exerc.* 1994;26(10):S271-S275.

9. Footman LG, Myerburg R. Sudden death in athletes: an update. *Sports Med.* 1998;26(5):335-350.

10. Cheitlin MD, Douglas PS, Parmley WW. 26th Bethesda Conference: recommendations for determining eligibility for competition in athletes with cardiovascular abnormalities, task force 2: acquired valvular heart disease. *Med Sci Sports Exerc.* 1994;26(10):S254-S260.

11. Graham Jr TP, Bricker JT, James FW, et al. 26th Bethesda Conference: recommendations for determining eligibility for competition in athletes with cardiovascular abnormalities, task force 1: congenital heart disease. *Med Sci Sports Exerc.* 1994;26(10):S246-S253.

12. Kaplan NM, Deveraux RB, Miller Jr HS. 26th Bethesda Conference: recommendations for determining eligibility for competition in athletes with cardiovascular abnormalities, task force 4: systemic hypertension. *Med Sci Sports Exerc.* 1994;26(10):S268-S270.

13. Maron BJ, Isner JM, McKenna WJ. 26th Bethesda Conference: recommendations for determining eligibility for competition in athletes with cardiovascular abnormalities, task force 3: hypertrophic cardiomyopathy, myocarditis, and other myopericardial diseases and mitral valve prolapse. *Med Sci Sports Exerc.* 1994;26(10):S261-S267.

14. Zipes DP, Garson Jr A. 26th Bethesda Conference: recommendations for determining eligibility for competition in athletes with cardiovascular abnormalities, task force 6: arrhythmias. *Med Sci Sports Exerc.* 1994;26(10):S276-S283.

15. Maron BJ. Cardiovascular risks to young persons on the athletic field. *Ann Intern Med.* 1998;129(5):379-386.

16. Anzai AK. Adolescent chest pain. *Am Fam Physician.* 1996;53(5):1682-1690.

17. VanCamp SP. Sudden death. *Clin Sports Med.* 1992;11(2):273-289.

18. Boissonnault WG, Bass C. Pathological origins of trunk and neck pain, part II: disorders of the cardiovascular and pulmonary systems. *J Orthop Sports Phys Ther.* 1990;12(5):208-215.

19. Bandy WD, Stong L, Roberts T, et al. False aneurysm—a complication following an inversion ankle sprain: a case report. *J Orthop Sports Phys Ther.* 1996;23(4):272-279.

20. Cohn SL, Taylor WC. Vascular problems of the lower extremity in athletes. *Clin Sports Med.* 1990;9(2):449-470.

21. Karas SE. Thoracic outlet syndrome. *Clin Sports Med.* 1990;9(2):297-310.

22. Rettig AC. Neurovascular injuries in the wrists and hands of athletes. *Clin Sports Med.* 1990;9(2):389-417.

23. Sotta RR. Vascular problems in the proximal upper extremity. *Clin Sports Med.* 1990;9(2):379-388.

24. Herbert PN, Hricik D. Inherited disorders of connective tissue. In: Andreoli TE, Carpenter CCJ, Plum F, et al, eds. *Cecil's Essential of Medicine.* 2nd ed. Philadelphia, Pa: WB Saunders Company; 1990:444-446.

25. McKeag DB. Preparticipation screening of the potential athlete. *Clin Sports Med.* 1989;8(3):373-397.

26. Bickley LS, Hoekelman RA. *Bates' Guide to Physical Examination and History Taking.* 7th ed. Philadelphia, Pa: Lippincott Williams & Wilkins; 1999.

27. DeGowin RL, Brown DD. *DeGowin's Diagnostic Examination.* 7th ed. New York: McGraw-Hill; 2000.

28. Smith AN, Bell GW. Hypertrophic cardiomyopathy and its inherent danger in athletics. *Athletic Training.* 1991;26(4):319-323.

29. Gould BE. *Cardiovascular and Lymphatic Disorders. Pathophysiology for the Health-Related Professions.* Philadelphia, Pa: WB Saunders Company; 1997:159-212.

30. Bryan G, Ward A, Rippe JM. Athletic heart syndrome. *Clin Sports Med.* 1992;11(2):259-272.

31. Miles WM, Zipes DP. Myocardial and pericardial disease. In: Andreoli TE, Carpenter CCJ, Plum et al, eds. *Cecil's Essentials of Medicine.* 2nd ed. Philadelphia, Pa: WB Saunders Company; 1990:105-112.

32. Garson AJ. Arrhythmias and sudden cardiac death in elite athletes. *Pediatr Med Chir.* 1998;20:101-103.

33. Tanji JL. Exercise and the hypertensive athlete. *Clin Sports Med.* 1992;11(2):291-302.

34. Dimeff RJ. Headaches in athletes. *Clin Sports Med.* 1992;11(2):339-349.

35. Palatini P. Exaggerated blood pressure response to exercise: pathophysiologic mechanisms and clinical relevance. *Journal of Sports Medicine and Physical Fitness.* 1998;38(1):1-9.

36. Frenkel EP. Anemias. In: Beers MH, Berkow R, eds. *The Merck Manual of Diagnosis and Therapy.* 17th ed. Whitehouse Station, NJ: Merck Research Laboratories; 1999:849-883.

37. Raunikar RA, Sabio H. Anemia in the adolescent athlete. *Am J Dis Child.* 1992;146:1201-1205.

38. Chatard J, Mujika I, Guy C, et al. Anemia and iron deficiency in athletes: practical recommendations for treatment. *Sports Med.* 1999;27(4):229-240.

39. Nichols AW. Nonorthopedic problems in the aquatic athlete. *Clin Sports Med.* 1999;18(2):395-411.

40. Jones JD, Kleiner DM. Awareness and identification of athletes with sickle cell disorders at historically black colleges and universities. *Journal of Athletic Training..* 1996;31(3):220-222.

41. Browne RJ, Gillespie CA. Sickle cell trait: a risk factor for life-threatening rhabdomyolysis. *The Physician and Sports Medicine.* 1993;21(6):80-88.

42. Harrelson GL, Fincher AL, Robinson JB. Acute exertional rhabdomyolysis and its relationship to sickle cell trait. *Journal of Athletic Training.* 1995;30(4):309-312.

43. Buzzard BM. Sports and hemophilia: antagonist or protagonist. *Clin Orthop.* 1996;328:25-30.

44. Nuber GW, McCarthy WJ, Yao JS, et al. Arterial abnormalities of the hand in athletes. *Am J Sports Med.* 1990;18(5):520-523.

45. Hoppenfeld S. *Physical Examination of the Spine and Extremities.* Norwalk, Conn: Appleton & Lange; 1976.

46. Magee DJ. *Orthopedic Physical Assessment.* 2nd ed. Philadelphia, Pa: WB Saunders Company; 1992.

47. Nesheiwat F, Sergi AR. Deep venous thrombosis and pulmonary embolism following cast immobilization of the lower extremity. *J Foot Ankle Surg.* 1996;35(6):590-594.

48. Alexander JK. Pulmonary embolism. In: Beers MH, Berkow R, eds. *The Merck Manual of Diagnosis and Therapy.* 17th ed. Whitehouse Station, NJ: Merck Research Laboratories; 1999: 593-601.

49. Goodman CC, Snyder TEK. Overview of cardiovascular signs and symptoms. In: Goodman CC, Snyder TEK, eds. *Differential Diagnosis in Physical Therapy: Musculoskeletal and Systemic Conditions.* 3rd ed. Philadelphia, Pa: WB Saunders Company; 2000:88-144.

50. Goodman CC. The respiratory system. In: Goodman CC, Boissonnault WG, eds. *Pathology: Implications for the Physical Therapist.* Philadelphia, Pa: WB Saunders Company; 1998:399-455.

51. Hallett JWJ. Diseases of the aorta and its branches. In: Beers MH, Berkow R, eds. *The Merck Manual of Diagnosis and Therapy.* 17th ed. Whitehouse Station, NJ: Merck Research Laboratories; 1999:1776-1784.

Pulmonary System

PURPOSES

- Describe the basic pulmonary structures and their functions.
- Review pathophysiological mechanisms of the pulmonary system.
- Describe the response of the pulmonary system to exercise.
- Discuss medical history results that are relevant to pulmonary pathology.
- Identify signs and symptoms of pulmonary pathology.
- Perform physical examination tasks relevant to the pulmonary system.
- Discuss, compare, and contrast selected pathological conditions of the pulmonary system.

Figure 4-1. Schematic representation of the lungs.

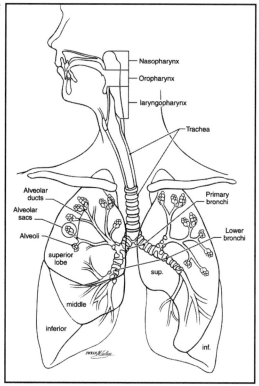

Introduction

The pulmonary system extracts oxygen from the air and exchanges it with carbon dioxide in the blood, thus performing a critical life-sustaining function.[1,2] Pulmonary disorders are the second most frequent cause of disability and the fifth leading cause of death among adults.[3] In addition, an estimated 14 to 15 million people have asthma, although their ability to participate in physical activity is not necessarily limited.[4] Chronic pulmonary diseases can be classified as either obstructive or restrictive.[4] Obstructive diseases (eg, asthma) limit air flow, whereas restrictive conditions (eg, from scoliosis) limit physical lung expansion.[4] Athletic trainers will encounter many persons with pulmonary disorders and should therefore be aware of the pathophysiology and signs and symptoms related to these conditions.

Review of Anatomy, Physiology, and Pathogenesis

The lungs, consisting of the bronchi, alveoli, and a rich blood supply, are the primary organs of the pulmonary system (Figure 4-1). Gases from the environment enter the nasopharynx, pass down the trachea, through the bronchi and bronchioles, and arrive in the alveoli. The capillary-rich alveoli, the terminal units of the respiratory pathway, exchange gases with the blood. The other airway structures are sometimes referred to as "dead space" since they do not participate in respiration (the physiological exchange of gases). In some pulmonary disorders, the amount of this physiological dead space in the lung increases and creates a functional (ie, nonanatomic) obstruction to respiration.[1] The upper airway (primarily the nasopharynx) adds warmth and moisture as it filters the incoming air.[1,2,5] Filtering is accomplished by mucus and tiny hair-like projections (cilia) that cover the upper airway and bronchi. Particles are trapped by the mucus and moved upward by the cilia to be expelled by coughing.

During the process called ventilation, air moves into and out of the lungs as an effect of changing pressures within the thorax. During inspiration, as the diaphragm and external intercostal muscles contract, the thorax expands in circumference. The visceral and parietal pleura maintain a negative pressure in the space between them and, thus, move the lung surface and thorax simultaneously. As the pressure inside the thorax falls below atmospheric pressure, the lungs expand and draw air in. Expiration of air occurs passively as alveolar pressure exceeds atmospheric pressure and elastic recoil of the ribcage compresses the lungs.[2,5]

Hence, inspiration requires active muscle contraction, whereas expiration occurs passively (although some muscles can cause forceful expiration).[2,5] Accessory inspiratory muscles include the abdominals, sternocleidomastoid, and scalenes. The levator scapulae and trapezius also participate in cases of severe respiratory distress. Accessory muscles of ventilation are not normally active during quiet breathing but become active as oxygen demand or the work of breathing increases.[5]

Oxygen and carbon dioxide are exchanged in the alveoli by a diffusion process called respiration (Figure 4-2). The rate of diffusion varies depending on the difference in partial pressures across the alveolar wall. Oxygen partial pressure in the atmosphere is greater than pressure in the alveolar capillaries, so oxygen moves into the blood across the single-celled walls of the alveoli.[1] Likewise, carbon dioxide moves into the alveoli since the partial pressure in the capillaries is greater than in the atmosphere.[1]

Many complex mechanisms affect gas exchange in the lung, as any standard physiology text will discuss in detail.[1] Essentially, when ventilation or lung blood flow is sufficiently disturbed, the process of binding oxygen and hemoglobin is impaired. Blood oxygen levels begin to fall rapidly when this occurs, which has severe physiological and metabolic consequences.

Breathing is regulated by several mechanisms. The first involves regions of the medulla oblongata that are sensitive to carbon dioxide and pH (a measure of chemical acidity and alkalinity) levels in the blood.[2,5] Carbon dioxide and most metabolic byproducts carried in the blood are acidic and thereby decrease blood pH. Stimulation of this breathing center causes increased ventilation rate and depth to expel acidic waste products.[1,5] Second, baroreceptors (sensitive to pressure) in the aorta and carotid arteries detect decreasing blood pressure. Chemoreceptors (sensitive to particular substances) in the same areas detect decreasing blood oxygen levels. These mechanisms combine to cause a reflex increase in ventilation to maintain blood oxygen concentration.[1,5]

Last, the nervous system regulates several processes related to breathing. Stretch receptors in the intercostal muscles cause inspiration to stop and expiration to begin.[5] Neurons controlling ventilation muscles (diaphragm, intercostal, and accessory muscles) travel through the phrenic nerve (from nerve roots C3 to C5), cranial nerve XI (sternocleidomastoid), and segmental thoracic nerves supplying the intercostal muscles.[5] Voluntary control of breathing is conducted through corticospinal tracts to the diaphragm and intercostal neurons.[1] Damage to the spinal cord above vertebral level C3 or C4 usually necessitates the use of a ventilator.

Figure 4-2. Diffusion of gases across the alveolar wall.

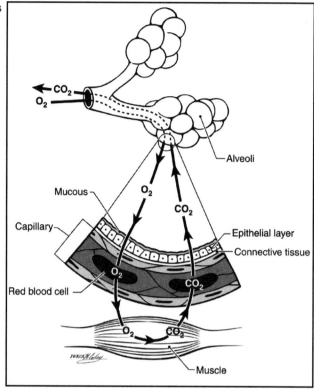

Both ventilation and respiration exhibit normal changes during exercise. First, the lungs receive increased blood as heart rate and stroke volume (ie, cardiac output) increases. Next, exercising muscles decrease the partial pressure of oxygen decreases in pulmonary blood. As a consequence, a higher proportion of the oxygen inhaled diffuses into the alveolar capillaries. Last, to meet the growing oxygen demand, rate of ventilation increases nearly immediately with the onset of exercise.[1]

Atelectasis is the collapse of a lung segment's alveoli, usually a result of a complete obstruction by an object or mucous lodged in the bronchi (Figure 4-3).[1] Atelectasis leads to pulmonary hypertension and cor pulmonale, and increases risk for development of pneumonia. Patients who are bedridden can develop atelectasis. In athletics, lung contusion from a severe blow to the thorax can cause atelectasis, which produces dyspnea, cough, and hemoptysis. Auscultation may detect diminished breath sounds or rales (see below) in the affected area. Depending on the amount of lung tissue damaged, full recovery or return to sports is gradual and can take quite some time.[6]

SIGNS AND SYMPTOMS

Dyspnea

Dyspnea (breathlessness or shortness of breath) occurs as blood oxygen levels decrease. Airway obstruction, metabolic imbalances, psychological stress (anxiety), mechanical restric-

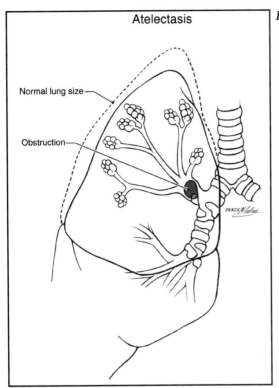

Atelectasis

Figure 4-3. Atelectasis.

Normal lung size

Obstruction

tion of the lungs, cardiac pathology, or pulmonary disease can cause dyspnea.[3,7] Healthy persons unaccustomed to high altitudes experience dyspnea since atmospheric oxygen is significantly lower than at sea level. Dyspnea produced by the supine position is called orthopnea. Orthopnea is caused by body fluids shifting to the lungs, enlarged abdominal organs pushing on the diaphragm, or left heart failure.[3,7]

Cough

A cough indicates irritation in the airway, which occurs with a variety of conditions.[8] A dry, nonproductive (no sputum) cough is most often caused by allergic reactions to environmental irritants.[3] A cough producing clear sputum suggests upper airway irritation. Purulent (containing pus) or opaque sputum may also indicate a lower respiratory infection.[3,7,9] Hemoptysis (cough with bloody sputum) is a sign of damaged lung tissue and requires prompt medical attention.[3,7-9]

Cyanosis

General, or central, cyanosis occurs when oxygen concentration in arterial blood decreases below 85%, causing a bluish tint in the fingernails, lips, and face.[3,7,8]

Figure 4-4. Pain patterns of pulmonary structures.

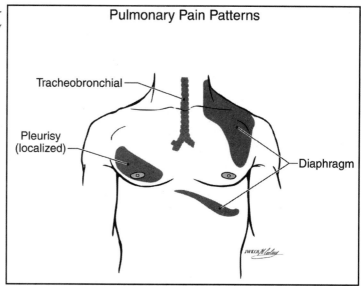

Pulmonary Pain Patterns

Tracheobronchial

Pleurisy (localized)

Diaphragm

Abnormal Breathing Pattern

Normal and abnormal breathing patterns may be described by rate, depth, effort, and pattern.[3] Normal breathing in adults is 10 to 15 breaths per minute, shallow (about 500 ml), relatively effortless, and regular. Children's breathing patterns are similar except more rapid (up to 20 breaths per minute). Changes in any of these parameters may suggest pulmonary impairment.

Thorax Pain

Chest pain over a specific lung lobe can be produced by pulmonary disorders.[2,3,8] Pulmonary structures can also cause pain in the back or side if the parietal pleura becomes irritated or inflamed.[3]

PAIN PATTERNS

Pain from pathology in the pulmonary system rarely occurs without accompanying signs and symptoms (coughing, wheezing, sore throat, dyspnea, etc).[10] Pulmonary structures can refer pain to the chest, neck, and shoulders, as seen in Figure 4-4.[2,10]

Lung

Tumors in the apex of the lung (Pancoast tumor) may compress the brachial plexus and vascular structures, causing pain and vascular symptoms (numbness, pallor, cramping) in the upper extremity.[10] Tumors can also compress on the bronchi, causing cough, dyspnea, or chest pain. Pain from lung tissue usually does not occur until inflammation affects the parietal pleura.[11]

Tracheobronchial

The trachea and proximal bronchial tree refer pain to the overlying cutaneous areas.[2]

Diaphragm

Diaphragmatic pain usually refers to the ipsilateral shoulder but may also occur in the neck, ribs, or spine.[2,8,10] Abdominal hemorrhage is characterized by a similar pain referral pattern resulting from irritation of the central diaphragm (see Chapter Five).[2]

Pleurisy

Pleural pain, or pleurisy, results from inflammation of the parietal pleura.[2,3,10] Inflamed pleura creates sharp, stabbing pain over the affected area and changes with coughing or deep inspiration.[3,7,8,10,11] Pleurisy can occur with trauma, infection, tumors, or pulmonary disease.[2,3]

MEDICAL HISTORY AND PHYSICAL EXAMINATION

Family and Personal History

Cigarette smoking is a strong risk factor for virtually all acquired pulmonary disorders.[10] In addition, a careful history can reveal a previously undetected chronic pulmonary disorder (intermittent symptoms with respiration, coughing, or sneezing) or infection (fever, recent infection, fatigue).[10] Blunt trauma to the chest or sudden deceleration may lead to lung injury.[12]

Symptoms

Dyspnea, cough, chest tightness, and decreased exercise capacity are common pulmonary symptoms. These symptoms may or may not be associated with activity or exercise and may change with deep breaths, speaking, or laughing.[2,4,13,14]

Inspection

The ribcage and spinal column should be examined for obvious deformities or asymmetry that affect inspiration, such as pectus excavatum (Figure 4-5a), pectus carinatum (Figure 4-5b), or scoliosis. Obesity can restrict ribcage expansion and diaphragm contraction, thus hindering the breathing mechanism.[9]

Palpation

In sitting or supine, the mechanics of breathing can be evaluated by palpating and observing the motion of the ribcage. Bilateral palpation should be done at the superior, anterior, inferior, and posterior aspects of the ribcage. With normal inspiration, the ribcage moves symmetrically and the ribs and abdomen rise together. Examples of abnormal patterns are the

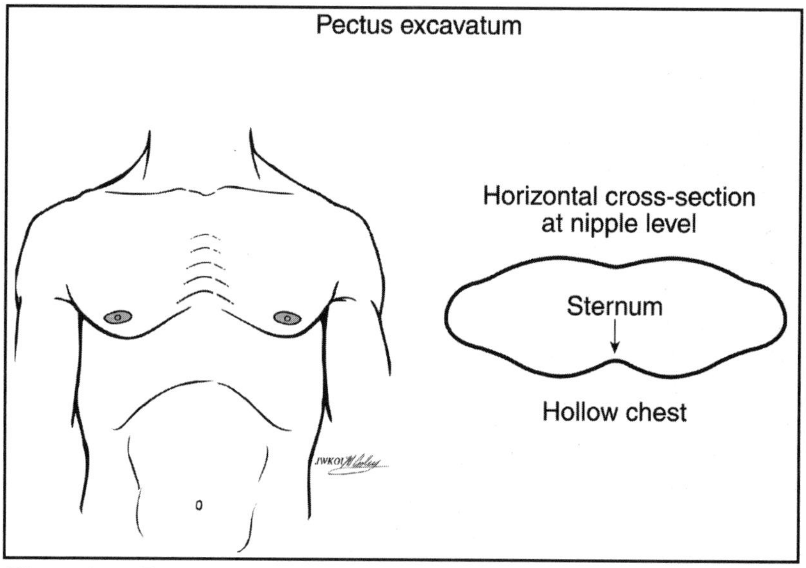

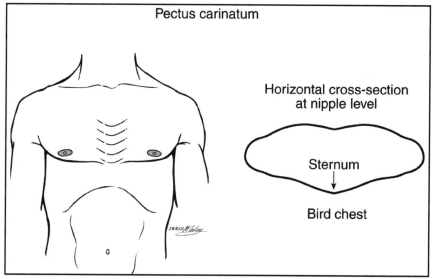

Figure 4-5a. Pectus excavatum.

Figure 4-5b. Pectus carinatum.

abdomen rising first, no movement of the ribcage, excessive use of accessory breathing muscles (sternocleidomastoid, abdominals, levator scapula, or trapezius), or asymmetrical expansion or contraction of the ribcage.[8] Palpation can also reveal crepitus (subcutaneous grinding sensation), which indicates air leaking into the subcutaneous tissues, or fremitus (vibration), suggesting pulmonary or pleural edema.[12]

Percussion

Lab Activity 4 (page 235) describes percussion relative to the pulmonary system. Alternating between contralateral sites allows comparison of percussion sounds.[9] Hyperresonance (sounding like a drum), indicates abnormal air space in the thorax, as occurs with pneumothorax.[12] Pulmonary or pleural edema produces a dull thud rather than the normal hollow sound over the lungs.[9] Areas of the thorax that do not sound normal to percussion should next be auscultated.[9]

Auscultation

Air passing through the stiff upper airway (trachea and bronchi) normally creates some turbulence, which can be auscultated. The soft alveoli, however, tend to dampen transmission of sound, so auscultated sounds are dull. Lab Activity 5 describes the process of pulmonary auscultation.[9,15]

Normal breath sounds, when heard outside their normal anatomical regions (Figure 4-6), are considered abnormal.[9] Normal tracheal and bronchial sounds are like wind rushing through a metallic tube, the bronchial sounds slightly more muffled. The expiratory phase is usually much louder than the inspiratory phase for both of these sounds. Vesicular breath sounds, described as "rustling leaves" and of a lower pitch than bronchial sounds, are heard over most of the thorax, with the inspiratory phase more prominent. Bronchovesicular sounds are similar to vesicular sounds upon inspiration and bronchial sounds upon expiration.[9]

Clearly heard spoken sounds (bronchophony), whispered sounds (whispered pectoriloquy), or high-pitched but intelligible spoken sounds (egophony) are all abnormal.[9] Inflammation of the pleura, obstruction of a bronchus, or atelectasis cause "decreased breath sounds," in which the normal breath sounds are less audible or absent.[8,9]

Abnormal auscultated sounds (adventitious sounds) include rales (crackles), rhonchi (wheezes), stridor, and pulmonary friction rub.[9] Rales, a series of distinct pops or cracks during inspiration, occur when blocked bronchi cause a collapse of distal bronchioles and alveoli (ie, atelectasis).[8,9] Rhonchi, continuous rumbling sounds during both inspiration and expiration, indicate an incomplete obstruction of bronchi or lower trachea that produces the distinctive sound of turbulent air.[8,9]

Stridor, a harsh, raspy sound that is audible upon inspiration (often without a stethoscope), suggests a sudden and nearly complete obstruction of the airway by a foreign object or inflammation.[9] Stridor that occurs while coughing is called croup.[7] A person with stridor, which is a medical emergency, should be closely monitored and immediately transported to a medical facility.

Last, when the visceral and parietal pleura become inflamed, a pleural "friction rub" can be auscultated. The friction rub sounds like creaking or clicking at the end of inspiration and is most commonly auscultated over the posterior and lateral thorax.[9] In addition, pain may cause the person to pause during inspiration and expiration.

Figure 4-6. Normal locations of auscultated breath sounds.

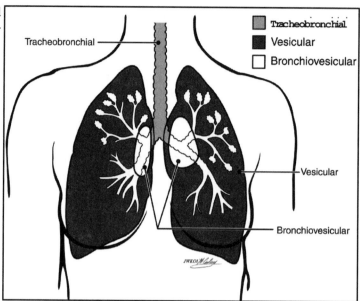

Respiration Rate and Depth

Normally, adults take between 12 and 15 breaths per minute. The relative length of inspiration and expiration is 1:1. The inspiratory and expiratory phases last approximately the same amount of time.[1] In persons with obstructive pulmonary disorders, however, the expiration phase is significantly longer than inspiration.[9]

An increased rate (over 20 breaths per minute) or depth (over 750 ml) of ventilation is called hyperpnea. When oxygen concentration in the blood decreases (hypoxemia), ventilation depth increases, but rate initially remains normal. Persons with metabolic hyperpnea (from hypoxemia) will eventually increase their rate of breathing as a chronic adaptation to low blood oxygen concentration. In contrast, an increase in breathing rate without an increase in depth, known as hyperventilation, rapidly decreases carbon dioxide concentration in the blood and increases pH (alkalosis).

Holding the breath can discern metabolic hyperpnea from hyperventilation. Persons with hyperpnea have difficulty holding their breath, which increases their hypoxemia, and their condition does not improve. Other pulmonary signs (cyanosis, chest pain) usually accompany this medical emergency. Hyperventilation, a common condition often caused by anxiety, improves when the breath is held, which allows carbon dioxide concentration and pH to return to normal. Hyperventilation is not an emergency.

Heart Rate

See Chapter Three.

Blood Pressure

See Chapter Three. As blood oxygen concentration decreases, hypertension occurs to maintain oxygen delivery to the tissues.[3]

Peak-Flow Meter (Hand-Held Spirometer)

A spirometer is an instrument used to measure lung volumes during ventilation. Spirometers typically found in athletic training environments are hand-held devices called peak-flow meters. As the subject expires into a small tube after taking a full inspiration, an analog scale or dial provides a measure of peak expiratory flow (PEF). PEF is an indication of airway function, which is affected by conditions such as asthma (acute bronchospasm and inflammation). Once a "personal best" PEF is established, peak-flow meter measures can be taken each day immediately before physical activity. For persons with moderate to severe asthma, a PEF less than 80% of personal best indicates impending acute bronchospasm (asthma attack). Prescribed medication may restore PEF. If not, participation in vigorous activity is contraindicated.[16]

PATHOLOGY AND PATHOGENESIS

Disorders of the Lung and Thorax

Drowning and Near-Drowning

Drowning causes many deaths among children, adolescents, and young adults.[3] Water aspiration (inhalation into the lungs) physically damages lung structures, causing atelectasis and infection.[3] In addition, the person may asphyxiate (die from failure of ventilation and respiration) from reflex spasm of the larynx.[3,17] Among near-drowning survivors, neurological and renal complications produce the most obvious and disabling physiological consequences. Time of immersion and temperature of the water determines the extent of tissue damage in these systems.

Anoxia (lack of oxygen) causes severe, irreversible neurological and renal damage within minutes. Cold water temperatures, however, allow longer immersion (particularly in children) due to the mammalian diving reflex, which reduces metabolic demand.[17] Hence, upon finding a potentially drowned person, begin and continue resuscitation efforts until advanced medical care is obtained. While 90% of those rescued while drowning survive, 20% have permanent complications. Rapid, progressive respiratory failure can occur 12 to 24 hours after a near-drowning incident, so all such victims should be transported to a hospital.[3]

Flail Chest Injury

A "flail chest" results from multiple rib fractures creating a free-floating segment of ribcage (Figure 4-7).[3] This region bulges upon expiration and collapses upon inspiration, referred to as "paradoxical excursion" of the chest. Flail chest injury is a medical emergency and is often accompanied by pneumothorax (see below).

Pulmonary Obstructive Disorders

Chronic Obstructive Pulmonary Disease

Chronic obstructive pulmonary disease (COPD) is a classification of diseases involving partially blocked airways. Examples of COPD include asthma, bronchitis, emphysema, and cystic fibrosis.[2,3,9,18] Obstruction caused by mechanical insufficiency, bronchospasm, or inflammation traps air in the lower airway, increasing residual volume (air remaining in the

Figure 4-7. Flail chest injury.

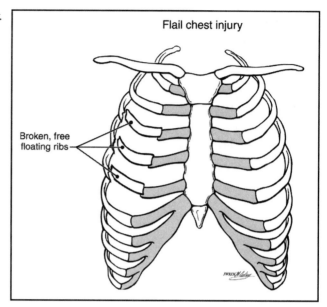

Flail chest injury

Broken, free floating ribs

lung) and decreasing the volume exchanged during ventilation (vital capacity). In the lungs, carbon dioxide concentration increases and oxygen concentration decreases, thus disrupting the diffusion gradient between the alveoli and capillaries and impairing gas exchange.[18] Asthma and exercise-induced bronchospasm are the COPDs most commonly encountered among athletes.

Asthma

Asthma, an abnormal autonomic regulation of bronchial muscles, produces bronchospasm, partial airway obstruction, chronic bronchial inflammation, and bronchial edema.[3,13,18,19] Asthma affects between 5% and 10% of the population, with both genetic and immune system factors.[3,19,20] Asthma causes intermittent acute bronchospasm, epithelial cell damage, and fibrous bronchiole changes. Airway obstruction occurs from a combination of inflammation and bronchospasm.[3,16,19,20]

Symptoms of acute bronchospasm include a sensation of chest constriction, sudden fatigue, and anxiety.[3,4,21] Clinical signs are dyspnea, inspiratory wheezing, prolonged expiration, and panting speech, which may also be accompanied by leaning forward (to assist breathing), cyanosis, and (in severe cases) seizure.[3,16] Hyperpnea and tachycardia occur as breathing becomes more difficult and hypoxemia increases.[3,16] Auscultation reveals decreased breath sounds and inspiratory rhonchi.[16]

Asthmatic bronchospasm may be precipitated by allergens (see Chapter Ten), infection, cold or dry air, drugs, and certain emotional states.[2,13,20] Goals of asthma treatment include limiting bronchial inflammation, controlling symptoms, preventing exacerbation, maintaining normal pulmonary function, and limiting side effects of medication.[19] Pharmacological treatments are classified into long-term control or acute relief medications, either of which can be inhaled or taken orally.[19] Anti-inflammatory medications are used for long-term control, whereas bronchodilatation medications provide quick relief from acute bronchospasm.

To manage an acute asthma attack, the person should sit, take deep breaths, exhale through pursed lips (to increase pressure throughout the airway), and attempt to remain emotionally calm.[21] Administration of an inhaler, if one has been prescribed, is indicated. Recovery should occur gradually in less than 1 hour.[3] Severe attacks that do not respond to these routine measures constitute an emergency. Asthma can produce pneumothorax, acute right heart failure, hypoxemia, and metabolic collapse.[3,16] The athletic trainer should be aware of the medications each athlete with asthma uses to control both chronic symptoms and acute attacks. Strict adherence to a prescribed medication regimen can prevent severe attacks.[3]

Exercise-Induced Bronchospasm

Exercise-induced bronchospasm (EIB) is more common than asthma, affecting approximately 15% of the population, 90% of people with asthma, and 35% to 40% of people with allergies.[13,22] EIB occurs 5 or 10 minutes into an exercise session and becomes progressively worse as activity continues. Spontaneous recovery occurs 30 to 60 minutes after stopping exercise.[4,13,14,22,23]

Cool or dry air and breathing through the mouth during vigorous exercise seem to exacerbate EIB.[14,22] Symptoms include unusual dyspnea and central chest pain during exercise.[4,13,14,22] Coughing after strenuous exercise occurs very commonly with EIB. Syncope and cyanosis may appear in severe cases.[4,13,14,22]

Preventative treatment involves control of underlying asthma (if present), medication, and environmental precautions (ie, avoiding cool, dry air).[3,4] In addition, prolonged warm-up (60 minutes before competition, exercise 10 to 15 minutes at 50% maximal heart rate, then rest 15 minutes before beginning full exercise session) to induce mild EIB and a refractory period.[14,22,23] If control cannot be obtained, switching sports or exercise in humid, warm environments may be indicated.[4] Bronchodilators, either oral or inhaled, effectively control EIB but have undesired side effects for physical activity (eg, anxiety, tremor, tachycardia). In addition, many of these medications are banned by competitive athletic associations.[14,22]

Acute EIB is managed much like acute asthma attack. Stop exercise, reassure the person emotionally, assess for anaphylaxis (see below), and monitor until symptoms resolve. EIB that persists for more than 60 minutes or produces syncope or cyanosis at any time is an emergency.

Exercise-Induced Anaphylaxis

A history of breathing problems during exercise combined with chronic use of nonsteroidal antiinflammatory drugs increase the risk of exercise-induced anaphylaxis (EIA), an abnormal immune response to vigorous physical activity.[22] EIA causes a "flush" sensation (heat in the head and neck) during exercise that is rapidly followed by coughing, stridor, and shock.[13] Skin lesions (urticaria or hives) 0.5 to 1 inch across may also appear.[22] Wheezing and other signs of bronchospasm are usually not present, but a resonant or barking-type cough (croup) may appear as the condition progresses.[22] Hypotension and tachycardia herald the onset of shock. Maintaining an airway, administering supplemental oxygen, and emergency transport are indicated. Intravenous medications (eg, adrenaline) are required to open the airway.[22]

Airway Inflammation

Bronchitis, rhinitis, and sinusitis all occur in the upper airway and can cause obstruction. Typically, allergic reactions (atopy) cause rhinitis, infections or allergies cause sinusitis, and infections or environmental irritants cause bronchitis.[3] See Chapter Nine for a discussion of upper respiratory infections.

Bronchitis

Acute bronchitis can result from infection or chemical irritation.[2,3] Early signs and symptoms include fever, nonproductive cough, sore throat, and musculoskeletal chest pain (from violent and persistent coughing).[2,3] Acute bronchitis progresses to a productive cough, wheezing, and systemic signs of infection. Cough suppressants, rest, and hydration are the usual course of treatment.[3] If neglected, the edema and irritation produced by acute bronchitis can progress to a severe bronchial infection.

Prolonged or repeated exposure to irritants causes chronic bronchitis, inflaming the bronchial mucous membranes.[2,3] The diameter of the bronchi decreases, thus impairing airflow. As distal bronchioles become completely obstructed, air is trapped in the alveoli, causing hypoxemia, cyanosis, and pulmonary hypertension. Right ventricular hypertrophy in response to increased pulmonary tension (cor pulmonale) forms peripheral edema.[3]

Wheezing and dyspnea are prominent, and fever may develop. A cough that is more productive in the mornings and evenings attempts to clear the airways.[3] A cough present 3 months a year for 2 consecutive years and accompanied by reduced expiratory capacity with no medical explanation suggests chronic bronchitis.[2,3,18]

Emphysema, a complication of chronic pulmonary disease and prolonged smoking, is not likely to be encountered in physically active persons.[18] Destruction of alveolar walls, and capillaries, and reduced lung elasticity decreases lung area available for gas exchange. Emphysema produces dyspnea, increased breathing effort, infection, and cor pulmonale.[2,3] The lung destruction in emphysema is irreversible and prognosis is very poor.

Restrictive Lung Disorders

Scarring of the lung from trauma, surgery, chemotherapy, or radiation can limit lung volume and, consequently, limit pulmonary function.[4] Physical activity is limited by impaired respiratory function and decreased capacity.[4]

Pneumothorax, Hemothorax, and Pneumomediastinum

Pneumothorax

Pneumothorax, or a "collapsed lung" from air in the pleural space, occurs either from sudden increase in lung pressure or trauma causing pleural injury.[1,3,6,12,24] The negative pressure normally in the pleural space is lost and the lung retracts instantly toward the bronchial tree (Figure 4-8). Without negative pleural pressure, the lung cannot inflate when the thorax expands.

Symptoms include acute pleuritic chest pain and dyspnea. Signs of hyperpnea, decreased or absent breath sounds upon auscultation, crepitus (palpable subcutaneous air in the thorax), and hyperresonance upon percussion may be noted over the affected lung.[3,6,12,24] If the pleural space continues to collect air with no mechanism to expel it, a tension pneumothorax results, in which the intrathoracic pressure rises rapidly with respect to the environment (Figure 4-9). The trachea and mediastinum (containing the heart) may deviate to one side and the thorax may twist asymmetrically.[3,6] If uncorrected, the pressure occludes the major vessels and compresses the heart, causing death. Treatment requires decompression with a chest tube inserted surgically through the thorax wall.

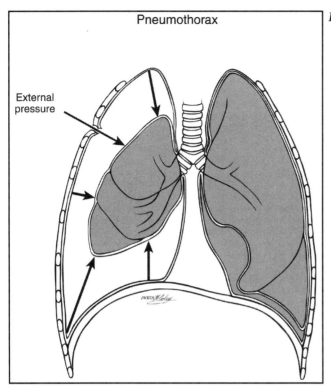

Pneumothorax

External pressure

Figure 4-8. Pneumothorax.

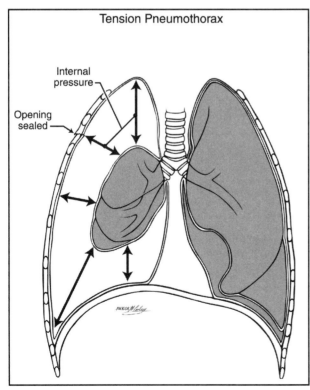

Tension Pneumothorax

Internal pressure

Opening sealed

Figure 4-9. Tension pneumothorax.

Figure 4-10. Hemopneumothorax.

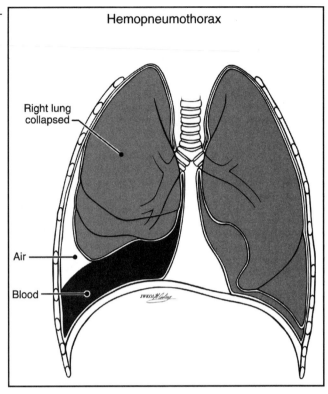

Hemopneumothorax

Right lung collapsed

Air

Blood

Hemothorax

If blood enters the pleural cavity, the condition is called hemothorax. The presence of both blood and air is a hemopneumothorax (Figure 4-10).[1,3] Signs and symptoms are similar to pneumothorax, but splashing can sometimes be auscultated in the lower lung lobes with changes in posture.

Suspected pneumothorax is treated by splinting the thorax by hugging a pillow, trying to control coughing or gasping for air, monitoring vital signs, and immediate emergency transport.[24] Returning to sports after pneumothorax (not tension or hemothorax) can occur within days of discharge from the hospital if other injuries (eg, rib fractures) permit.[6] Tension pneumothorax, hemopneumothorax, and pneumothorax with concomitant traumatic injuries require more extensive medical care and a longer course of recovery.

Pneumomediastinum

Air can also spontaneously leak into the mediastinum (the anatomic space between pulmonary compartments), referred to as pneumomediastinum. Spontaneous pneumomediastinum occurs after a forceful effort that increases pressure in the thorax (eg, Valsalva's maneuver, cough, or sneeze).[25] Asthma, diabetes, illicit drug use, anorexia nervosa, and pulmonary disorders are significant risk factors for this condition.[25] Chest pain similar to pneumothorax appears but is localized to the sternum rather than the lateral thorax. Neck pain or difficulty swallowing (dysphagia) may also be reported.[8,25] Pneumomediastinum is usually not an emergency, usually resolving within 10 days unless a more serious condition (eg, pulmonary embolism, pneumothorax) coexists. Physical activity can be gradually resumed if symptoms are absent and the condition does not recur.[25]

PEDIATRIC CONCERNS

Cystic Fibrosis

Cystic fibrosis (CF) is the most commonly inherited disorder among caucasian Americans.[3,4,26] The genetic abnormality affects the exocrine glands, primarily in the respiratory system and digestive tract.[2,3,26] Thick secretions of these glands block the airway, which tends to become infected.[2,4,18] Pneumonia (bacterial pulmonary infection; see Chapter Ten) is recurrent, progressively disabling, and eventually fatal. Only half of people with CF live to 30 years of age.[3,4,18,26] Treatment includes nutritional support, regular pulmonary hygiene to clear secretions, and antibiotic medications.[3,4,18,26] Mild- to moderate-intensity exercise is recommended to improve aerobic fitness, survival time, and function.[4]

Neuromotor Disease

Respiratory disability often accompanies chronic neuromuscular diseases (see Chapter Eight) that affect the respiratory muscles or neural control of breathing.[4] In addition, chest wall deformities, either congenital or acquired, can restrict lung volumes and thus impede pulmonary function.[4] Deformities of the thorax; such as pectus excavatum, pectus carinatum, and scoliosis, should be referred for medical examination to rule out underlying cardiac or congenital disorders.[4]

Persons with scoliosis are not restricted from sports participation unless the curve is progressing rapidly, prohibits trunk movement, or limits ventilation.[4] Sports participation for persons who have had surgical spinal fixation to correct scoliosis depends on residual pulmonary impairment and limitations of the surgical hardware or trunk strength and motion.[4]

SUMMARY

The pulmonary system exchanges oxygen and carbon dioxide (respiration) between the body and the environment by inspiring and expiring air (ventilation). Dyspnea, cough, cyanosis, thoracic chest pain, and abnormal breathing patterns are the most common signs and symptoms of pulmonary pathology. Percussion and auscultation are used to assess potential pulmonary disorders. Pulmonary pathology can occur in the lung tissue (trauma, drowning) as obstructive conditions (asthma, bronchospasm), restrictive disorders (trauma or surgical scarring, infection, deformity), or collapse of interpleural space (pneumothorax, hemothorax, pneumomediastinum).

RESOURCES

Auscultation (Pulmonary)

- UCLA School of Medicine auscultation assistant site with audio of breath sounds. www.med.ucla.edu/wilkes/index.htm

- Virtual Stethoscope site with audio of breath sounds (McGill University). www.music.mcgill.ca/auscultation/auscultation.html

Pulmonary

- American Lung Association. www.lungusa.org
- atlife.com pulmonary site. www.atpulmonary.com/pulm
- Yahoo directory. dir.yahoo.com/Health/Diseases_and_Conditions/Respiratory_Diseases

REFERENCES

1. Ganong WF. *Review of Medical Physiology.* 15th ed. Norwalk, Conn: Appleton & Lange; 1991.

2. Goodman CC, Snyder TEK. Overview of pulmonary signs and symptoms. In: Goodman CC, Snyder TEK, eds. *Differential Diagnosis in Physical Therapy: Musculoskeletal and Systemic Conditions.* 3rd ed. Philadelphia, Pa: WB Saunders Company; 2000:145-180.

3. Goodman CC. The respiratory system. In: Goodman CC, Boissonnault WG, eds. *Pathology: Implications for the Physical Therapist.* Philadelphia, Pa: WB Saunders Company; 1998:399-455.

4. Homnick DN, Marks JH. Exercise and sports in the adolescent with chronic pulmonary disease. *Adolescent Medicine.* 1998;9(3):467-481.

5. Dantzker DR, Tobin MJ. Anatomical and physiological considerations. In: Andreoli TE, Carpenter CCJ, Plum F, et al, eds. *Cecil's Essentials of Medicine.* 2nd ed. Philadelphia, Pa: WB Saunders Company; 1990:126-135.

6. Amaral JF. Thoracoabdominal injuries in the athlete. *Clin Sports Med.* 1997;16(4):739-753.

7. Loudon RG. Approach to the pulmonary patient. In: Beers MH, Berkow R, eds. *The Merck Manual of Diagnosis and Therapy.* 17th ed. Whitehouse Station, NJ: Merck Research Laboratories; 1999: 511-521.

8. Dantzker DR, Tobin MJ. Approach to the patient with respiratory disease. In: Andreoli TE, Carpenter CCJ, Plum F, et al, eds. *Cecil's Essentials of Medicine.* 2nd ed. Philadelphia, Pa: WB Saunders Company; 1990:124-126.

9. Arnall D, Ryan M. Screening for pulmonary system disease. In: Boissonnault WG, ed. *Examination in Physical Therapy Practice: Screening for Medical Disease.* 2nd ed. New York: Churchill-Livingstone; 1995: 69-100.

10. Boissonnault WG, Bass C. Pathological origins of trunk and neck pain, part II: disorders of the cardiovascular and pulmonary systems. *J Orthop Sports Phys Ther.* 1990;12(5):208-215.

11. Stopka CB, Zambito KL. Referred visceral pain: what every sports medicine professional needs to know. *Athletic Therapy Today.* 1999;4(1):29-36.

12. Kizer KW, MacQuarrie MB. Pulmonary air leaks resulting from outdoor sports: a clinical series and literature review. *Am J Sports Med.* 1999;27(4):517-520.

13. Mellman MF, Podesta L. Common medical problems in sports. *Clin Sports Med.* 1997;16(4):635-662.

14. Virant FS. Exercise-induced bronchospasm: epidemiology, pathophysiology, and therapy. *Med Sci Sports Exerc.* 1992;24(8):851-855.

15. Bickley LS, Hoekelman RA. *Bates' Guide to Physical Examination and History Taking.* 7th ed. Philadelphia, Pa: Lippincott, Williams & Wilkins; 1999.

16. Ellis EF. Asthma. In: Beers MH, Berkow R, eds. *The Merck Manual of Diagnosis and Therapy.* 17th ed. Whitehouse Station, NJ: Merck Research Laboratories; 1999:556-568.

17. Dean NL. Near drowning. In: Beers MH, Berkow R, eds. *The Merck Manual of Diagnosis and Therapy.* 17th ed. Whitehouse Station, NJ: Merck Research Laboratories; 1999:2459-2460.

18. Dantzker DR, Tobin MJ. Obstructive lung disease. In: Andreoli TE, Carpenter CCJ, Plum F, et al, eds. *Cecil's Essentials of Medicine.* 2nd ed. Philadelphia, Pa: WB Saunders Company; 1990:140-147.

19. Jain P, Golish JA. Clinical management of asthma in the 1990s: current therapy and new directions. *Drugs.* 1996;52(6):1-11.

20. Spahn JD, Szefler SJ. The etiology and control of bronchial hyperresponsiveness in children. *Curr Opin Pediatr.* 1996;8:591-596.

21. Arnheim DD, Prentice WE. Other health conditions related to sports. In: Arnheim DD, Prentice WE, eds. *Principles of Athletic Training.* 8th ed. St. Louis, Mo: Mosby-Year Book; 1993:796-819.

22. Kyle JM. Exercise-induced pulmonary syndromes. *Sports Med.* 1994;78(2):413-421.

23. Nichols AW. Nonorthopedic problems in the aquatic athlete. *Clin Sports Med.* 1999;18(2):395-411.

24. Cvengros RD, Lazor JA. Pnuemothorax: a medical emergency. *Journal of Athletic Training.* 1996;31(2):167-168.

25. Ferro RT, McKeag DB. Neck pain and dyspnea in a swimmer: spontaneous pneumomediastinum presentation and return-to-play considerations. *The Physician and Sports Medicine.* 1999;27(10):67-71.

26. Rosenstein BJ. Cystic fibrosis. In: Beers MH, Berkow R, eds. *The Merck Manual of Diagnosis and Therapy.* 17th ed. Whitehouse Station, NJ: Merck Research Laboratories; 1999:2366-2371.

Chapter Five

Gastrointestinal and Hepatic-Biliary Systems

PURPOSES

- Describe the basic gastrointestinal and hepatic-biliary structures and their functions.
- Review pathophysiological mechanisms of the gastrointestinal and hepatic-biliary systems.
- Describe the response of the gastrointestinal and hepatic-biliary systems to exercise.
- Discuss medical history findings relevant to gastrointestinal and hepatic-biliary pathology.
- Identify signs and symptoms of gastrointestinal pathology.
- Identify signs and symptoms of hepatic-biliary pathology.
- Perform physical examination tasks relevant to the gastrointestinal and hepatic-biliary systems.
- Discuss, compare, and contrast selected pathological conditions of the gastrointestinal and hepatic-biliary systems.

INTRODUCTION

Intensity and duration of exercise can alter the functions and mechanical digestive processes of the gastrointestinal (GI) system. Thus, GI symptoms (nausea, vomiting, abdominal pain, diarrhea, constipation) are common in athletes.[1,2] In addition, GI problems are very frequent in the general population. For instance, over 10% of people are affected by irritable bowel syndrome (discussed later) and consequently experience GI symptoms almost daily.[2]

Trauma, infection, and disease can affect the organs of the GI system (esophagus, stomach, small and large intestines), producing very similar signs and symptoms regardless of etiology. GI infections will be discussed in Chapter Ten. Pathological conditions of the liver and gallbladder (hepatic-biliary system), both of which are intimately related to the GI system, are included in this chapter. Trauma to GI organs and the abdomen are rare in sports but are also difficult to recognize and can have grave consequences.[3,4] Any athlete who sustains significant trauma to the abdomen should thus be examined and monitored closely.[4] This chapter reviews physical examination of the abdomen and signs and symptoms of common gastrointestinal and hepatic-biliary pathology.

REVIEW OF ANATOMY, PHYSIOLOGY, AND PATHOGENESIS

The structures and organs of the GI system include the mouth, esophagus, stomach, small intestine (duodenum, jejunum, and ileum), large intestine, rectum, and anus (Figure 5-1). The functions of the upper GI system (from the mouth through the duodenum) are to ingest (take in) and digest (chemically break down) food. The lower GI system (from the jejunum through the rectum) absorbs nutrients and water, and eventually expels waste products of digestion.[5,6] Figure 5-2 shows the abdominal quadrants and the organs contained by these imaginary boundaries. Remembering the location of anatomical structures within each quadrant is important when examining the abdomen.

Gastric emptying accelerates with the onset of exercise.[2,7] Once exercise intensity reaches about 75% of aerobic capacity, however, gastric emptying slows.[2,7] Gastric emptying during exercise is aided by avoiding fatty foods before exercise and consuming cool, dilute liquids.[2,7] Overall, lower GI (bowels) motility increases with regular exercise.[2] Since gravity assists the GI system, upright activity increases bowel motility in persons who have been immobile. During exercise, however, small intestine motility apparently slows as a result of transient ischemia and exercise-induced hormone release.[7] Furthermore, movement of the large bowel in the gut during exercise may cause diarrhea or mild abdominal cramping.[4,7] Proper hydration can prevent many of these exercise-induced GI symptoms.[2]

The liver, gallbladder, and exocrine pancreas each secrete digestive enzymes into the duodenum through the same opening (ampulla of Vater). In addition, the liver receives the blood from the intestines, colon, spleen, and pancreas before it returns to the heart. This blood flow pathway allows the liver to absorb nutrients and catabolize toxins. In addition, the liver regulates metabolism of fats and cholesterol and stores large amounts of carbohydrate. It also forms bile, which contains salts that emulsify fat and pigments (eg, bilirubin) during digestion. Most bile salts are recycled through the GI-hepatic circulation, whereas the pigments are excreted, giving feces its distinctive coloring.

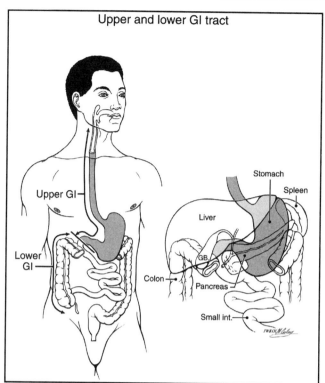

Upper and lower GI tract

Figure 5-1. Organs of the upper and lower gastrointestinal system.

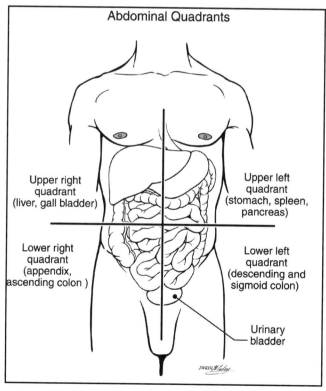

Abdominal Quadrants

Figure 5-2. Abdominal quadrants and their contents.

Bile flows into the duodenum when food is present. Otherwise, it is stored and becomes more concentrated in the gallbladder. Disorders of the biliary (liver and gallbladder) system produce high levels of bilirubin, a yellow pigment, in the blood, which leads to jaundice (yellow discoloration) of the skin, eyes, and mucosa. In addition, digestion and absorption of fats is impaired from the subsequent lack of bile salts in the small intestine.

The pancreas consists of two functional segments. The endocrine pancreas, discussed in Chapter Seven, secretes hormones (insulin and glucagon) that regulate blood carbohydrate levels. The exocrine pancreas secretes several enzymes important to digestion of carbohydrates, proteins, and fats. Diseases affecting the exocrine pancreas can thus produce substantial digestive impairment. In addition, insufficient secretion of pancreatic enzymes, which are highly alkaline to counter the acidity of gastric juices, has been associated with development of duodenal ulcers.[8]

Signs and Symptoms

Nausea and Vomiting

Nausea and vomiting (emesis) are hallmarks of upper GI disorders. Nausea and vomiting occur when nerve endings in the upper GI are irritated by chemical, mechanical, or autonomic (vagus nerve) stimuli.[2,5,9] When blood appears in vomitus, the condition is called hematemesis. A person with nose or mouth trauma may accidentally swallow and then vomit bright red blood. If blood collects in the stomach, as occurs with pathological upper GI bleeding, the vomitus appears like coffee grounds.[5] Gastric ulcers, excessive use of nonsteroidal anti-inflammatory drugs (or other drugs), alcohol abuse, or major systemic illness can produce upper GI bleeding.[5] Rarely, intense exercise can also cause acute gastric hemorrhage and hematemesis.[7]

Abdominal Pain

Location (ie, specific abdominal quadrant), severity, and quality of abdominal pain should be noted. Description of the pain may aid in discerning affected structures or likely pathology. Severe, progressive cycles of intense cramping-type pain (called *colic*) is produced by acute inflammation or obstruction of an abdominal organ or duct.[10] Acute, localized, constant pain indicates inflammation of the parietal peritoneum (peritonitis).[10] Nontraumatic, mild abdominal cramps usually indicate lower GI disorders.[2,11] Notably, nonsteroidal anti-inflammatory medications may temporarily eliminate GI pain.[9]

Abdominal Rigidity

Protective spasm of the muscular abdominal wall is called *rigidity*. Rigidity is detected during palpation as hardness rather than the normal suppleness of the abdomen. Rigidity usually occurs in a specific quadrant or region rather than the whole abdomen. Significant abdominal pain and difficulty flexing the trunk accompanies rigidity. Abdominal rigidity requires immediate medical attention.

Loss of Appetite and Significant Loss in Body Weight

Loss of appetite (anorexia) can be indicative of upper GI problems.[2,9] A significant loss of body weight suggests poor nutritional absorption, dehydration from recurrent vomiting or diarrhea, or increased metabolic demand of chronic disease.[5] More ominously, infection and cancer each induce loss of appetite and weight loss.[2] Cancer will be discussed in Chapter Eleven.

Night Pain or Symptoms

Abdominal symptoms that wake a person at night are nearly always serious. The parasympathetic nervous system, which is more active at night, stimulates the GI organs and produces symptoms as function of the affected organ increases.

Prandial or Postprandial Symptoms

Prandial (while eating) and *postprandial* (after eating) symptoms suggest GI or biliary pathology.[5,9,11] Stomach pain begins about an hour after eating, whereas duodenal pain occurs 2 hours or more after a meal. Food exacerbates a gastric ulcer but may relieve a duodenal ulcer.[9,11] In addition, caffeine, alcohol, and spicy foods may irritate gastroesophageal reflux or peptic ulcer. Fatty foods may exacerbate gallbladder or pancreas pathology.[6]

Change in Bowel Habits or Stool Quality

Changes in the frequency, regularity, or ease of defecation indicate lower GI pathology.[6,9] Changes in consistency, odor, or color of stool (feces) suggest disease in the lower GI or biliary systems.[6] Two disturbances of bowel habit are diarrhea and constipation.

Diarrhea describes frequent or loose bowel movements from increased bowel motility, malabsorption syndromes, infection, or a combination of these factors.[5,12,13] Increased urgency or diarrhea also occasionally occurs with vigorous exercise.[1,2] Some medications and drugs cause temporary diarrhea. For instance, antibiotics allow overproduction of intestinal bacteria (causing colitis), which increases intestinal motility.[5]

Constipation is abnormal retention of feces as a result of hardened (dehydrated) stool or decreased bowel motility.[5,11,12] Poor diet (high sugar, low fiber), dehydration, medications (eg, analgesics), stress, inactivity, or GI disease can contribute to constipation.[5,11] Chronically retained stool becomes impacted, causing a bowel obstruction that requires surgery.[11] Appropriate lifestyle changes relieve constipation due to diet or inactivity, although laxatives may be needed in more severe cases.

Rectal Blood

Bleeding from the rectum, either bright red or detected in the feces (hematochezia), heralds lower GI pathology.[1,9] Simple causes include hemorrhoids or anal fissures, but a physician is required to rule out irritable bowel syndrome, cancer, or parasitic GI infection.[1,7,11] Black, tar-like stools, called melena, suggest upper GI bleeding.[11]

Jaundice

Jaundice, or icterus, is yellow discoloration of skin, eyes, and mucous membranes occurring with excess bilirubin levels. Pathology of the liver, gallbladder, exocrine pancreas, or the

Figure 5-3a. Referred pain patterns for the upper gastrointestinal system.

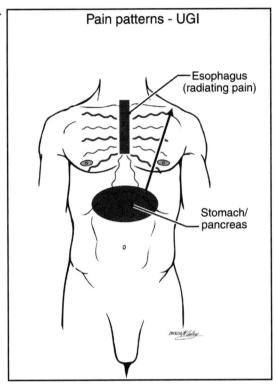

Pain patterns - UGI

Esophagus (radiating pain)

Stomach/ pancreas

common bile duct for these organs cause jaundice.[8] The urine progressively darkens and the stool progressively lightens in color as bilirubin increases in the blood (filtered by the kidneys into the urine) and decreases in the bowel.[9,11]

PAIN PATTERNS

Upper Gastrointestinal System

Referred pain from the upper GI (Figure 5-3a) may mimic that of the heart (see Chapter Three), but history and accompanying signs and symptoms usually clarify the system of origin.[2,7] The esophagus causes substernal pain, although occasionally pain is also noted in the epigastrium or radiating to the back.[5,7,9,11] Epigastric pain is produced by the stomach but may refer to the back or shoulder if the diaphragmatic pleura becomes irritated.[9,11,14]

Lower Gastrointestinal System

Pain from the small and large intestines present diffuse middle to lower abdominal pain (Figure 5-3b).[9,11,14]

Appendix

The appendix classically produces midabdominal pain that migrates to the right lower quadrant, one-third to one-half the distance from the anterior superior iliac spine toward the

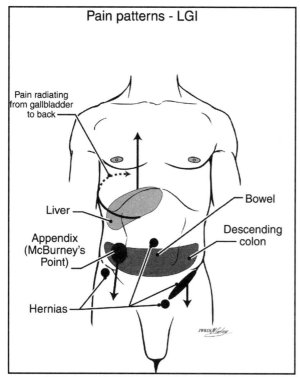

Figure 5-3b. Referred pain patterns for the lower gastrointestinal system.

umbilicus (McBurney's point).[9,11,14] Pain from acute appendicitis may also radiate to the central abdomen, hip, thigh, or lower back.[11]

Liver

The liver refers pain to the epigastrium and right upper quadrant, and can refer pain to the right shoulder, thoracic, or cervical spine if the inferior diaphragm is irritated.[9,11,14]

Gallbladder

The gallbladder produces a characteristic pattern along the right T8 dermatome, radiating to the right scapula as a sharp, stabbing sensation.[9,14] Gallbladder pain may begin as a sensation of heartburn.[11]

Pancreas

The pancreas produces epigastric pain that refers to the mid or lower back.[11] If the diaphragm becomes irritated, pain occurs in the left shoulder.[11]

MEDICAL HISTORY AND PHYSICAL EXAMINATION

Family and Personal History

A complete GI history should be conducted for any person reporting nausea, vomiting, or abdominal pain as a primary complaint.[2] Recent GI illness, change in diet, current training regimen, and recent travel can be related to the etiology of GI pathology.[1] Childhood diseases, recent surgery, current medications, and history of a similar condition should (as always) be ascertained.[10]

Symptoms produced at night or while eating are usually more serious than postprandial heartburn or exercise-induced indigestion.[2,9] Regular use of caffeine, alcohol, nicotine, drugs, or medications should be noted.[6,9]

Direct trauma can damage internal organs, including those of the GI and hepatic-biliary systems.[4] A history of very recent trauma to the abdomen or thorax may be more important than the current presentation of symptoms or signs, which may not indicate the severity of the injury for hours.[3] Trauma from the end of a blunt instrument (bicycle handlebars, baseball bat) or that produces bruising or rib fractures should raise suspicion of internal organ damage. Last, sudden deceleration of the thorax can cause the contents of the abdomen to collide with the ribcage, thus causing injury.[3]

Significant injuries to the liver, jejunum, or colon are rare in sports. Progressive deterioration of vital signs (shock) and persistent abdominal pain are serious signs. Symptoms should be assessed regularly for several hours following abdominal trauma.[4]

Inspection

A symmetric but abnormally protruding abdomen indicates ascites (excess peritoneal fluid), bowels distended by obstruction, or excessive gas in the bowels.[10] The abdomen may also appear asymmetric, usually indicating ascites (that shift with gravity), hepatomegaly (right enlargement), or splenomegaly (left enlargement).[6]

Other signs may be observable by close inspection. Small, bulging masses in the lower abdomen may be herniated bowel, particularly if tender or manually reducible. Pulsing may be observed with an aortic or iliac artery aneurysm (see Chapter Three).[10] Jaundice may be noted in the skin or sclera of the eyes. Severe abdominal muscle spasms cause a characteristic flexed or sidelying "fetal" posture, with both arms crossed over the belly.

Examination of the Abdomen

Lab Activity 6[4,6,10,15] outlines basic physical examination of the abdomen, including auscultation, percussion, and palpation. Differentiating musculoskeletal trauma, such as fractured ribs or strained abdominal muscles, from abdominal organ trauma or pathology can be difficult. Contraction of the abdominal muscles (by having the athlete raise the head in supine) may worsen musculoskeletal symptoms but virtually eliminate painful palpation of visceral pathology.[6] In addition, placing the left hand flat on the quadrants or over specific abdominal organs and striking briskly with the ulnar edge of the right fist (hammering) produces pain in injured organs.[15]

Manually depressing the abdomen on either the same or opposite side as the symptoms and quickly releasing the pressure is a test for rebound tenderness. Pain produced by this maneuver is suggestive of peritonitis.[4,6,16] Another test for detecting peritonitis is the "jar" test, also known as Markle's sign.[17] The person stands on his or her toes and drops suddenly to his or her heels. A sharp increase in abdominal pain is positive for peritonitis.[16]

Initial physical examination may not suggest intra-abdominal injury, thus requiring repeated examinations.[4] Almost half of emergency room patients with abdominal pain who have an initially negative physical examination actually have significant abdominal injuries.[2,4] Hence, the first indication of a declining condition after such an abdominal injury requires emergency transportation.

PATHOLOGY AND PATHOGENESIS

Upper Gastrointestinal Disorders

Dyspepsia

Burning pain in the chest, nausea and vomiting, and loss of appetite are the hallmarks of upper GI pathology.[2] The most common upper GI condition is dyspepsia, also known as indigestion or heartburn—an uncomfortable burning sensation under the sternum.[5,13] Irritation in the upper GI from medications, drugs, alcohol, caffeine, or nondisease states such as pregnancy cause dyspepsia.[5,13] This term also describes symptoms common to many GI disorders, including gastroesophageal reflux, peptic ulcer, and liver disease.[13] Signs such as weight loss, abnormal masses in the abdomen, hematochezia, or fever, however, do not occur with benign dyspepsia. Dyspepsia can usually be successfully managed with dietary changes or over-the-counter medications.

Gastroesophageal Reflux

Gastroesophageal reflux occurs when the esophageal sphincter malfunctions after ingestion of certain types of foods, medications, or drugs (caffeine, alcohol). Symptoms are produced by acid from the stomach entering the esophagus. Gastroesophageal reflux causes symptoms similar to dyspepsia.[5] Exercise involving repeated vertical impact forces, such as running, can also induce gastroesophageal reflux.[7] Third, psychoemotional stress stimulates the vagus nerve, causing excess stomach acid and stomach contractions that may push acid into the esophagus.[5] Most often, gastrointestinal reflux can be controlled with dietary and lifestyle changes (stress management) and use of antacids. If the condition prevents participation in physical activity, persists for several weeks, or becomes significantly worse, the athlete should be referred to a physician. Occasionally, prescribed medication is needed, as is surgery in rare instances.[7]

Peptic Ulcer

Peptic ulcer occurs when the gastric juices digest the submucosal layers of the stomach or duodenum.[5,6] Chronic infection by helicobacteri pylori (H. pylori) has been strongly associated with development of peptic ulcers.[18] Ulceration into the muscular layer produces scarring and erosion beyond the muscular layer and can perforate blood vessels, causing severe gastric hemorrhage.[5]

A peptic ulcer classically produces intermittent pain in the upper or middle abdomen that radiates to the thoracic spine, chest, and neck.[5,6,9] The symptoms often consistently improve or worsen after eating and may disappear and recur over several weeks or months. Abdominal pain at night is very common. If the condition persists, recurrent vomiting and loss of appetite cause weight loss.[6] A perforated ulcer may produce bloody vomitus (hematemesis), coffee-grounds vomitus, or melena.[5,6] Acute perforation can also cause shock and may require surgery.[18]

Peptic ulcers are most common among people who are elderly, taking nonsteroidal anti-inflammatory medications (eg, for arthritis), or using nicotine and alcohol heavily. Ulcers can occur, however, in physically active persons who are under psychological and physiological stress.[5,6] Avoidance of foods known to irritate the condition and use of antacids usually provide symptomatic relief.[18] Antibiotics and acid-reducing medications often succeed in healing peptic ulcers, although some patients (5% to 10%) experience recurrence. Only a few ulcers require surgery, usually for perforation with excessive bleeding or suspected malignancy.[18]

Gastritis and Gastroenteritis

Gastritis describes stomach inflammation that results from erosion of the entire mucosa, chronic use of medications (nonsteroidal anti-inflammatory drugs), H. pylori infection, or autoimmune diseases.[5,6] Gastritis can be acute or chronic, erosive or nonerosive. Acute erosive gastritis occurs in patients with severe chronic illness. Chronic erosive gastritis is most commonly attributable to nonsteroidal anti-inflammatory drugs, alcohol abuse, irritable bowel disease (see below), or viral infection.[18] Nausea, vomiting, and vague upper abdominal pain may be present in such cases. Dietary restrictions and symptomatic treatment with antacids are used as treatment, although recurrences are frequent.

Acute and chronic nonerosive gastritis is frequently a result of H. pylori infection, potentially causing gastric irritation, mucosa breakdown, peptic ulcers, and cancer.[18] Symptoms, when present, are similar to erosive gastritis and peptic ulcer. Treatment with antibiotics eliminates the bacteria and the condition.

Gastroenteritis is the inflammation of the mucosal lining of the stomach and intestines, usually a result of infection.[12,19] Food poisoning, traveler's diarrhea, and viral "stomach flu" are common manifestations of gastroenteritis, as discussed in Chapter Ten.

Lower Gastrointestinal Disorders

Cardinal signs of lower GI (jejunum, colon, and rectum) pathology are persistent diarrhea or hematochezia. Most commonly, infection causes diarrhea that resolves with simple supportive interventions (ie, hydration) within 5 days.[13] The medical history may reveal a pattern of similar illness among family or teammates, indicating an infectious origin. In such cases, the affected athletes should be temporarily isolated from teammates to prevent cross-contamination.

Radical changes in diet, excessive alcohol consumption, mechanical vibration from running long distances, and psychoemotional stress can also cause temporary diarrhea. An athlete with diarrhea should be withdrawn from participation until the syndrome resolves to prevent dehydration and proper, hydrated weight is restored.

Occasionally, diarrhea is the chief compliant in a person with more serious pathology, particularly if notably unusual in color or odor, or accompanied by fever, vomiting, or severe abdominal cramps. Recurrent or persistent diarrhea, particularly leading to weight loss or accompanied by other systemic signs and symptoms (fever, fatigue, etc), requires urgent referral to a physician for a diagnostic examination.[1]

Inflammatory Bowel Diseases

Inflammatory bowel diseases (Crohn's disease and ulcerative colitis) are genetic autoimmune disorders. The small intestine and colon initiate an immune reaction against their own cells, causing widespread ulceration, fibrosis, and necrosis.[5,11,20] Onset of the disease is usually in adolescence or early adulthood and coexisting immune disorders are common.[5] Inflammatory bowel diseases have a varied clinical presentation, including abdominal pain, chronic diarrhea, hematochezia, weight loss, palpable abdominal mass (particularly in the right lower quadrant), loss of appetite, skin rash, and intermittent joint pain.[5,11,20]

A key to recognition is the chronic recurrence of signs and symptoms. Inflammatory bowel diseases are not curable but can be medically managed with diet, lifestyle changes, medication, and surgery as needed.[5] Persons with diagnosed inflammatory bowel disease should be monitored during physical activity to maintain hydration. Exacerbation of symptoms are common. Approximately 30% of patients with ulcerative colitis and 70% of patients with Crohn's disease will require surgery.[20] Most will lead relatively normal, active lives if managed appropriately.

Irritable Bowel Syndrome

A similar but less severe and far more common condition is irritable bowel syndrome, thought to be a reaction to psychophysical stress and poor diet.[21] Irritable bowel syndrome produces abdominal pain and cramping, and is most prevalent among young adult females.[5,11,21] This disorder affects motility of the intestines, causing diarrhea, constipation, or alternating episodes of both. Bloating or abdominal distention may also appear. Relief of abdominal pain usually occurs after defecation.[21]

The course of irritable bowel syndrome is intermittent and usually recurrent but does not cause inflammation in the bowels, which distinguishes it from other disorders.[5] In addition, irritable bowel syndrome rarely interrupts sleep.[21] Stress reduction, dietary changes, and reasonable physical activity are the usual course of treatment.[11] Alcohol, nicotine, and caffeine use should be curtailed, and a physician should review current medication use. Medication may be prescribed to assist with stress or relieve symptoms.[5,21] With appropriate treatment, most affected people are not substantially limited by irritable bowel syndrome.

Appendicitis

The appendix lies in the lower right quadrant where the terminal ileum becomes the ascending colon. When the appendix becomes acutely inflamed by physical irritants or infection, a general, progressively increasing epigastric abdominal pain appears and eventually migrates to the lower right quadrant. McBurney's point becomes exquisitely sensitive, and rebound tenderness or a positive "jar sign" is present (see Lab Activity 5). Passive extension or active flexion of the right hip may be painful if the psoas muscle is also irritated.[15] Loss of appetite and nausea are usually present, although vomiting is rare.[3] Other signs of infection may be present, such as fever and malaise.

The usual treatment is surgical removal of the appendix, although nonsurgical medical treatment is sometimes successful. Return to activity after surgery occurs at 1 to 2 weeks in children and 3 to 4 weeks in adults (because of their larger surgical wound).[3] A ruptured appendix spills infected contents into the peritoneal cavity and is therefore much more serious. Early recognition and proper early management of appendicitis are key to prevention of rupture.

Figure 5-4. Location of indirect, direct, and femoral hernias.

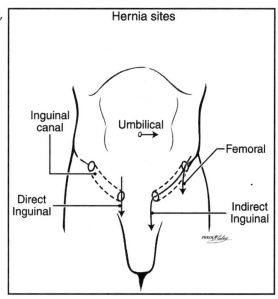

Hernia sites

Inguinal canal

Umbilical

Femoral

Direct Inguinal

Indirect Inguinal

Diverticulosis and Diverticulitis

Multiple herniations of the mucosa and submucosa of the intestine through the muscular layer of the intestinal wall is a condition called diverticulosis.[5] Ten percent of Americans and as many as half of the elderly population have this anatomical disorder.[5] In most cases, however, diverticulosis is asymptomatic.

When feces becomes trapped in a herniated section or a section becomes obstructed, diverticulitis (inflammation of the herniated section) results. Symptoms include severe abdominal cramping and constant pain in the lower left quadrant that may radiate to the back.[6] Additional signs include alternating constipation and diarrhea, fever, and rectal bleeding. Pain and cramps usually worsen a few hours after eating and may briefly resolve after defecation.[5] Treatment with a high-fiber diet and light exercise to encourage bowel motility is common. In more severe cases involving infection or complete bowel obstruction (causing an ischemic bowel segment), antibiotics and emergency surgery may be required.[5]

Hernia

Herniation occurs when an organ or part of an organ protrudes through a defect in the tissue that normally contains that organ.[5,6,22] A segment of small intestine can herniate into the inguinal canal, into the femoral canal (which contains the neurovascular bundle) under the inguinal ligament, or through the linea alba near the umbilicus (Figure 5-4). Inguinal, femoral, and umbilical hernias often cause a palpable bulge at the herniation.[3,5,6] With an indirect inguinal hernia, the herniated segment travels down the inguinal canal and into the scrotum, where the bowel loop may be palpated by the athlete during showering or self-examination. History may include a sudden tearing sensation upon exertion (although most will not remember a particular episode). Many hernias are detectable only by medical imaging and may be completely asymptomatic.[3,6]

With any type of hernia, the primary symptom is a burning pain in the groin. This pain worsens with activity, increase in abdominal pressure (Valsalva's maneuver), or body position.[5,6] Pain from an inguinal or femoral hernia may radiate into the anterior thigh, and an umbilical hernia produces pain in the abdominal wall. The intestinal segment may herniate only intermittently, causing inconsistent symptoms. A large, irreducible herniation requires surgical repair.[5,6] Modern surgical techniques allow laproscopic hernia repair. Gradual return to physical activity can be expected in about 1 week.[3] Open surgical repair necessitates an additional week or two of recovery.[3]

Hemorrhoids

Hemorrhoids, also called "piles," are varicose (dilated) veins in the rectum or anus. Internal hemorrhoids occur inside the rectum, whereas external hemorrhoids protrude through the anal border. In either case, bright red blood may appear with defecation, although no pain occurs unless the rectum or anus is fissured (split in tissue) or the veins become strangulated (ischemic).[5] Pain and itching accompany external hemorrhoids, particularly during sitting.

Very common and usually not medically serious, hemorrhoids can be quite bothersome. They are treated with changes in diet to soften the stool and reduce constipation, and topical medications to relieve symptoms. Occasionally, surgery is needed.

Abdominal Trauma

Persistent abdominal pain, localized tenderness, rigidity, or upper GI signs (nausea, vomiting, etc) after a blow to the ribs or abdomen requires emergency referral. If an athlete sustains a blow that fractures ribs, causes abdominal bruising, causes abdominal cramping, or produces rigidity, a physician should examine them as soon as possible.[3] In sports, the most commonly injured abdominal organs are the spleen and liver.

Spleen Trauma and Splenomegaly

The spleen stores platelets and other types of blood cells and filters the blood to remove small particles and deformed or old red blood cells. The spleen lies beneath the ninth to the 11th ribs and may thereby be injured by a direct blow to the left upper quadrant (LUQ).[3] Associated symptoms and signs include shock, nausea, vomiting, LUQ rigidity, abdominal pain, and referred pain in the left shoulder (also known as Kehr's sign).[2,3] Occasionally, signs of serious injury to the spleen appear very gradually and are difficult to recognize. Any suspicion of splenic injury (by history, symptoms, and existing signs) requires immediate withdrawal from participation and medical referral.

People with splenomegaly (pathological enlargement of the spleen, often from medical conditions such as mononucleosis; see Chapter Nine) require at least 3 weeks after onset before resuming physical activity and 1 month (or more) before returning to strenuous activity.[2,13] Splenomegaly greatly increases risk of acute splenic rupture, so athletes should obtain physician clearance before returning to contact or collision sports.[2,3]

Liver Trauma

Trauma to the liver progresses more slowly than does trauma to the spleen.[2,3,23] Persistent abdominal pain, right upper quadrant (RUQ) tenderness, and upper GI signs (nausea, vomiting, etc), however, warrant an emergency medical examination.[3,23] Many liver injuries do not require surgery but should be monitored overnight in a hospital and followed closely by a physician upon discharge.[3,4,23] Recovery from either surgical or nonsurgical treatment can take weeks or months.[23] A liver injury severe enough to require surgery often results in permanent exclusion from sports.[3]

Hepatic-Biliary Diseases

Hepatitis

Hepatitis, literally "inflammation of the liver," occurs primarily with viral infection or liver toxicity. Viral hepatitis types (A, B, C, D) refer to the different hepatitis viruses that directly attack the liver.[5,24] Hepatitis A virus is transmitted through close personal contact (oral-oral route; see Chapter Nine) or through contaminated food when preparers do not wash their hands properly after using the restroom (oral-fecal route). Hepatitis B, C, and D require direct exposure to body fluids (blood, urine, feces, saliva, mucous, tears, vomit, semen, or vaginal secretions).[24,25] Children and adolescents usually acquire hepatitis A, whereas young adults contract types B and C. Hepatitis D occurs as a complication of type B. Hepatitis B and C cause more severe liver damage than do A or D.[5]

Vaccines are available for hepatitis viruses A and B. Health care workers are at increased risk for contracting viral hepatitis since they are exposed to many people with chronic illness.[6] Thus, handwashing and strict adherence to standard precautions (ie, gloves, mask, and gown as needed) are mandatory in all health care environments.[24,25]

Generally, three stages of hepatitis infection are evident: initial, icteric, and recovery. The initial stage may not produce symptoms, although the hepatitis virus is highly communicable during this time.[11,24] During this stage, general systemic signs and symptoms appear and worsen in severity, including fatigue, loss of appetite, nausea, diarrhea, weight loss, and joint pain.[6,11] As hepatitis progresses, the urine darkens and stool lightens in color as bilirubin increases in the blood.[6,24] The liver becomes acutely enlarged and tender to palpation.

Three or 4 weeks after infection, the icteric stage produces jaundice that lasts 6 to 8 weeks, but the systemic signs slowly resolve.[5] Near the end of this stage, the liver begins to return to normal size, but the spleen enlarges and cervical lymph nodes may swell.[11] Interestingly, the virus is not communicable at this point. During the recovery stage, which takes 4 months or longer, fatigue is the most prominent symptom.[5,11,24]

Specific medical treatments do not exist for hepatitis, although antiviral agents and supportive measures are usually administered. Practicing infection control measures (rigorous handwashing when working with food or between patient contacts) and inoculating health care workers may prevent the spread of hepatitis. Most people infected with hepatitis A recover fully. Recovery from the other types of hepatitis depend on aggressiveness of infection and timing of medical intervention. Hepatitis B can be fatal.

Toxic hepatitis occurs with exposure to certain chemicals or drugs, including antibiotics, oral contraceptives, psychotropics, and cytotoxic drugs used to treat cancer.[11] The chemicals damage liver cells, which become necrotic. Symptoms and signs depend on the extent of necrosis. Clinical presentation resembles viral hepatitis, including jaundice, fatigue, loss of appetite, dark urine and light stools, fever, joint pain, and RUQ pain. Treatment is removal of the offending agent and avoidance of the toxin from that point forward.[5]

Chronic hepatitis can develop from viral infection, chronic exposure to toxins, or by unknown etiology.[5,24] Chronic hepatitis produces liver necrosis and cirrhosis (see below). Many secondary syndromes develop, such as arthritis, kidney disorders, and anemia. Chronic hepatitis is treated with steroids, which have many complications and side effects. Prognosis is poor.

Cirrhosis

Cirrhosis, the result of chronic liver disease and malnutrition, produces cellular damage and necrosis, which lead to fibrotic changes in the liver. The fibrous tissue eventually interferes with the liver's vascular supply and function, leading to ascites, splenomegaly, central and peripheral neurological signs, and GI system signs and symptoms.[11] Cirrhosis is not curable and does not heal. Medical treatment includes addressing the underlying cause (eg, alcohol abuse or hepatitis) to prevent further necrosis and supportive measures. Chronic hepatitis and cirrhosis often require a liver transplant.

Alcohol abuse is the leading cause of liver disease in America.[6,11] Prolonged consumption of large amounts of alcohol leads to hepatitis, cirrhosis, hepatic failure, and death. Cessation of alcohol intake in such cases is critical but is often very difficult both physically and psychologically. Chapter Eight discusses the psychological aspects of alcohol abuse.

Gallstones and Gallbladder Disease

Gallstones (cholelithiasis) and gallbladder disease (cholecystitis) both produce intermittent RUQ pain that worsens after meals that include fatty foods.[9] Gallstones account for nearly 20% of all hospital admissions among adults.[11] Increased risk of gallstones is associated with age, obesity, high-cholesterol diet, and diabetes.[9,11] Females are at higher risk, most likely because of elevated estrogen levels (as occurs during pregnancy, with oral contraceptive use, or in women who have had many children).[9,11]

Cholecystitis results when gallstones block the cystic duct (the gallbladder's attachment to the common bile duct). Fever, jaundice, vomiting, RUQ tenderness, and referred right shoulder pain suggest an acute gallbladder attack.[6,11] Chronic cholecystitis may present severe RUQ pain, accompanied by intolerance for foods high in fat or spice, heartburn, belching, constipation, or diarrhea.[9,11] Laproscopic surgery can remove the gallstones and thus relieve symptoms. Recovery depends on the size and extent of gallstones.

Pancreatitis

Acute pancreatitis occurs when pancreatic enzymes become active within the pancreas rather than the duodenum, resulting in self-digestion of pancreatic cells.[26] This cascades into a severe peritonitis, sudden and excruciating epigastric and LUQ pain, left shoulder pain, LUQ rigidity, and possibly shock. Infection can lead quickly to septicemia (bacteria in the bloodstream) and death. Acute pancreatitis is a medical emergency, with a dramatic clinical presentation of severe illness.[26]

SUMMARY

Many GI disorders can be attributed to lifestyle, including diet, nicotine and alcohol use, and physical inactivity. More serious disorders are caused by infection, chronic disease processes, or obstruction of the GI tract or ducts. Common signs and symptoms of gastrointestinal disorders include nausea, vomiting, diarrhea, constipation, and abdominal pain. The liver, gallbladder, spleen, and exocrine pancreas produce upper abdominal pain that may refer into either shoulder. Pathology of these organs are usually accompanied by disturbances in digestion. Medical emergencies of the abdomen, containing the GI system, hepatic-biliary system, and spleen, often produce peritonitis, recognizable by abdominal pain, tenderness, localized rigidity, and positive rebound or jar signs. Peritonitis causes fever or shock as it progresses, thereby demanding immediate medical care.

RESOURCES

Gastrointestinal

- The Acute Abdomen, a site instructing evaluation of acute abdominal pain (North Carolina State University and the Bowman Gray School of Medicine). www4.ncsu.edu/eos/users/w/wes/homepage/SIMS/Module2/GE2_4.html
- atlife.com gastrointestinal site. www.atgastroenterology.com/gi
- Yahoo directory. dir.yahoo.com/Health/Diseases_and_Conditions/Intestinal_Diseases

Hepatic-Biliary

- Diseases of the Liver (Departments of Medicine, Anatomy, and Cell Biology, College of Physicians & Surgeons, Columbia University). cpmcnet.columbia.edu/dept/gi/disliv.html
- Hepatitis Information Network; the Liver. www.hepnet.com/liver/index.html
- Yahoo directories:

  dir.yahoo.com/Health/Diseases_and_Conditions/Gall_Bladder_Disease/

  dir.yahoo.com/Health/Diseases_and_Conditions/Liver_Diseases/

REFERENCES

1. Butcher JD. Runners' diarrhea and other intestinal problems of athletes. *Am Fam Physician.* 1993;48(4):623-627.
2. Green GA. Gastrointestinal disorders in the athlete. *Clin Sports Med.* 1992;11(2):453-470.
3. Amaral JF. Thoracoabdominal injuries in the athlete. *Clin Sports Med.* 1997;16(4):739-753.
4. Ryan JM. Abdominal injuries and sport. *Br J Sports Med.* 1999;33(3):155-160.
5. Goodman CC. The gastrointestinal system. In: Goodman CC, Boissonnault WG, eds. *Pathology: Implications for the Physical Therapist.* Philadelphia, Pa: WB Saunders Company; 1998:456-495.
6. Koopmeiners MB. Screening for gastrointestinal system disease. In: Boissonnault WG, ed. *Examination in Physical Therapy Practice: Screening for Medical Disease.* 2nd ed. New York: Churchill-Livingstone Inc.; 1995:101-116.
7. Moses FM. The effect of exercise on the gastrointestinal tract. *Sports Med.* 1990;9(3):159-172.
8. Ganong WF. *Review of Medical Physiology.* 15th ed. Norwalk, Conn: Appleton & Lange; 1991.
9. Boissonnault WG, Bass C. Pathological origins of trunk and neck pain, part I: pelvic and abdominal visceral disorders. *J Orthop Sports Phys Ther.* 1990;12(5):192-207.
10. Stone R. Primary care diagnosis of acute abdominal pain. *Nurse Pract.* 1996;21(12):19-20, 23-26, 28-30, 35-41.
11. Goodman CC, Snyder TEK. Overview of hepatic and biliary signs and symptoms. In: Goodman CC, Snyder TEK, eds. *Differential Diagnosis in Physical Therapy: Musculoskeletal and Systemic Conditions.* 3rd ed. Philadelphia, Pa: WB Saunders Company; 2000:260-286.
12. Arnheim DD, Prentice WE. Other health conditions related to sports. In: Arnheim DD, Prentice WE, eds. *Principles of Athletic Training.* 8th ed. St. Louis, Mo: Mosby-Year Book; 1993:796-819.

13. Mellman MF, Podesta L. Common medical problems in sports. *Clin Sports Med.* 1997;16(4):635-662.

14. Stopka CB, Zambito KL. Referred visceral pain: what every sports medicine professional needs to know. *Athletic Therapy Today.* 1999;4(1):29-36.

15. Bickley LS, Hoekelman RA. *Bates' Guide to Physical Examination and History Taking.* 7th ed. Philadelphia, Pa: Lippincott, Williams & Wilkins; 1999.

16. DeGowin RL, Brown DD. *DeGowin's Diagnostic Examination.* 7th ed. New York: McGraw-Hill; 2000.

17. George B, Markle IV. A simple test for intraperitoneal inflammation. *Am J Surg.* 1973;125:721-722.

18. Finn S, Hirschowitz BI. Gastritis and peptic ulcer disease. In: Beers MH, Berkow R, eds. *The Merck Manual of Diagnosis and Therapy.* 17th ed. Whitehouse Station, NJ: Merck Research Laboratories; 1999:245-255.

19. Boyce TG. Gastroenteritis. In: Beers MH, Berkow R, eds. *The Merck Manual of Diagnosis and Therapy.* 17th ed. Whitehouse Station, NJ: Merck Research Laboratories; 1999:283-292.

20. Sachar DB, Walfish J. Inflammatory bowel diseases. In: Beers MH, Berkow R, eds. *The Merck Manual of Diagnosis and Therapy.* 17th ed. Whitehouse Station, NJ: Merck Research Laboratories; 1999:302-311.

21. Olden K. Functional bowel disorders. In: Beers MH, Berkow R, eds. *The Merck Manual of Diagnosis and Therapy.* 17th ed. Whitehouse Station, NJ: Merck Research Laboratories; 1999: 312-317.

22. Bickley LS, Hoekelman RA. *Bates' Guide to Physical Examination and History Taking.* 7th ed. Philadelphia, Pa: Lippincott, Williams & Wilkins; 1999.

23. Ray R, Lernire JE. Liver laceration in an intercollegiate football player. *Journal of Athletic Training.* 1995;30(4):324-326.

24. Simon JB. Hepatitis. In: Beers MH, Berkow R, eds. *The Merck Manual of Diagnosis and Therapy.* 17th ed. Whitehouse Station, NJ: Merck Research Laboratories; 1999:377-385.

25. Buxton BP, Daniell JE, Buxton BHJ, et al. Prevention of hepatitis B virus in athletic training. *Journal of Athletic Training.* 1994;29(2):107-112.

26. Freedman SD. Pancreatitis. In: Beers MH, Berkow R, eds. *The Merck Manual of Diagnosis and Therapy.* 17th ed. Whitehouse Station, NJ: Merck Research Laboratories; 1999:269-274.

Chapter Six

Renal and Urogenital Systems

PURPOSES

- Describe the basic renal and urogenital structures and their functions.
- Review pathophysiological mechanisms of the renal and urogenital systems.
- Describe the response of the renal and urogenital systems to exercise.
- Discuss medical history findings relevant to renal and urogenital pathology.
- Identify signs and symptoms of renal pathology.
- Identify signs and symptoms of urogenital pathology.
- Perform physical examination tasks relevant to the renal and urogenital systems.
- Discuss, compare, and contrast selected pathological conditions of the renal and urogenital systems.

Figure 6-1. Organs of the renal system and urinary tract.

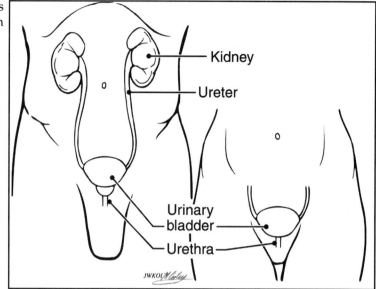

INTRODUCTION

The renal-urinary system, which includes the kidneys, ureters, bladder, and urethra (Figure 6-1), filters the blood, regulates extracellular fluid level, and eliminates metabolic waste from the blood and body.[1,2] The kidneys remove waste products and excess water from the blood. These substances are collected and sent through the ureters to the bladder and exit the body through the urethra as urine.[1,2] The kidneys contribute to homeostasis by providing hormonal and osmotic (fluid balance) control of BP, regulation of red blood cell production, and calcium regulation.[1-4]

Normal urine contains water, byproducts of protein metabolism (urea, creatine, and various acids), and salt (sodium chloride). It may also contain small amounts of glucose, dead cells, crystallized salts, and mucus. Blood cells and whole proteins should not be present in urine since their size normally prohibits absorption through the renal system.[4] The detection of protein during urinalysis is always pathological.

The kidneys can be damaged by trauma, toxins, chronic disease, and chronically abnormally high concentrations of glucose, urea, or creatine in the blood.[4] Kidney pathology affects vascular absorption at the nephron (the functional unit of the kidney).[4] Simply stated, as the filtering process changes, the kidney either extracts elements from the blood that it should not, fails to extract elements it should, or both. This results from the osmotic pressure in kidney capillaries (glomeruli) becoming more like the osmotic pressure in the blood. Consequently, the nephron absorbs a large amount of fluid in an effort to restore proper osmotic tension. The increased fluid, however, affects the ability of the kidney to draw solutes (waste products) into the urine.

Over time, metabolic byproducts collect in the blood and cause damage to other systems, notably the cardiovascular and neurological systems. Since the kidneys play a critical role in regulation of blood pressure, hypertension is often a consequence of chronic kidney disorders. In addition, disturbance of acid-base balance produces metabolic imbalances (acidosis or alkalosis) that depress or excite the central nervous system.

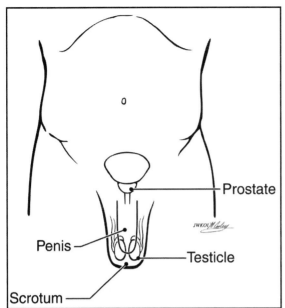

Figure 6-2. Organs of the male genital system.

Prostate

Penis

Testicle

Scrotum

The male genital (reproductive) system includes the prostate gland, the spermatic cord, the testicles and associated organs of spermatozoa production, the urethra, and the penis (Figure 6-2). The female genital system includes the ovaries, fallopian tubes, uterus, and vagina (Figure 6-3). Some organs of the genital system are stimulated by hypothalamus and pituitary hormones to release the gender-specific hormones testosterone (from the testes) and estrogen (from the ovaries). These "sex hormones" induce puberty (development of sexual maturation and secondary sex characteristics) and regulate sexual health and function.[2]

Trauma, infection, tumors (Chapter Nine), hormonal imbalances (Chapter Seven), and congenital conditions can produce pathology of the genital systems in both males and females. This chapter includes discussions of gender-specific medical conditions that affect physical activity. Pathology of the female breast, although not technically part of the urogenital system, will be discussed in this chapter.

REVIEW OF ANATOMY, PHYSIOLOGY, AND PATHOGENESIS

The kidneys have a dual role in the control of BP, both of which are linked by a single mechanism. First, the kidneys secrete the hormone renin, which indirectly increases vascular resistance (vasoconstriction) and consequently increases BP. Second, elimination of excess fluid through the kidney maintains a consistent fluid level in the body.[3,5]

If fluid level drops, as occurs with severe bleeding or dehydration, BP initially decreases. When BP decreases (for any reason), renin is released, which constricts the blood vessels and increases BP. Conversely, if the kidney is unable to excrete excess fluid or the blood retains excess fluid (hypervolemia), BP rises since the volume of fluid in the closed vascular system exerts increased pressure on the vascular walls.[3] With chronic secretion of renin or hyperv-

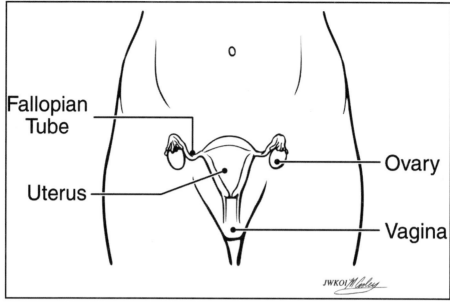

Figure 6-3. Organs of the female genital system.

olemia, systemic hypertension results. Chronic hypertension, whether caused by hormonal or fluid imbalances, damages the nephrons of the kidney.

During resistance exercise, systolic and diastolic BP increases in proportion to exercise load. Thus, persons with cardiovascular or kidney problems are advised to avoid resistance training. During endurance exercise, however, systolic BP increases moderately, levels off, and then gradually decreases back to normal as exercise continues. Diastolic BP changes very little during any stage of endurance exercise. Endurance exercise thus contributes to control of hypertension and is therefore recommended for persons with pathology of the cardiovascular or renal systems, or who have hypertension.

The organs of the pelvis, including the genital systems of both genders, are supported by a horizontal sling of muscles.[6] These muscles suspend the organs within the pelvic cavity and assist in urinary and sexual function. Impaired function of these muscles can contribute to urinary or sexual disability, even in the absence of any other pathology.

Several hormones from the hypothalamus regulate menstruation, which prepares the uterine lining (endometrium) for implantation of a fertilized ovum and regularly sloughs the lining if implantation does not occur (Figure 6-4). The hypothalamic hormones also stimulate the pituitary gland to release hormones that affect estrogen and progesterone production in the ovaries.[7,8]

Estrogen and progesterone interact to produce endometrial development in the presence of ovulation, the release of an ovum from the ovaries that occurs approximately 2 weeks before menses.[6] When estrogen and progesterone levels decrease, the thick, blood-rich endometrium is expelled (menses) to prepare the uterus for the next cycle. The menstrual cycle is very sensitive to hormonal levels and nutrition. Amenorrhea (absence of menses), a very common finding among female athletes, occurs with pregnancy (implantation of a fertilized ovum), endocrine disorders, or malnutrition.

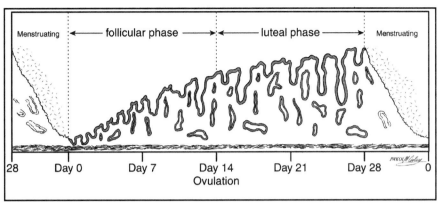

Figure 6-4. Menstruation.

Signs and Symptoms

Hematuria

Blood in the urine is either a sign of kidney or bladder pathology, or a side effect of prolonged strenuous exercise. Gross hematuria after a blow to the back or abdomen suggests kidney, ureter, or bladder injury, and is a medical emergency. Infection of the kidney or bladder produces subtle hematuria accompanied by the signs and symptoms discussed in Chapter Nine.

Exertional or "sports" hematuria develops from either exercise-induced renal ischemia during long duration, high-intensity exercise, or repetitive microtrauma of the kidney or bladder during running or other vigorous activity.[9] Treatment is rest, medical referral, and gradual return to activity. Activity can resume 24 hours after urine returns to normal.[9]

Sexual Dysfunction

Impotence, painful intercourse, blood in the semen (hemospermia), unusual bleeding during intercourse, or loss of libido (psychoemotional sex drive) are symptoms of urogenital pathology. Individuals reporting these symptoms should be encouraged to see a physician.

Menstrual Irregularities

Amenorrhea and other changes in the menstrual cycle can occur with pathology of the female reproductive system. Amenorrhea is most commonly caused by pregnancy but may occur with dietary restriction, hormonal imbalances, or exercise excesses among athletes. Amenorrhea in young, healthy females is not normal and requires medical evaluation.[10] Characteristically, adolescents display wide variation in regularity and intensity of menses.

PAIN PATTERNS

Kidneys, Ureters, and Bladder

Kidneys refer pain to the ipsilateral lower back or abdomen, or cause general lower abdominal pain.[11,12] Ureters usually cause severe pain in the groin, thigh, and abdomen.[11,12] Bladder pain occurs in the suprapubic region with referral to the lower back or thighs.[11,12]

Obstruction in the upper urinary tract (kidney or ureter) produces acute intermittent pain in the abdomen and unilateral lower back that radiates to the ipsilateral lower abdominal quadrant, groin, or perineum.[1] Lower urinary tract obstruction (bladder, urethra) produces an aching pain in the lower abdomen.[1]

Male Urogenital System

Testicular trauma produces a distinctive, temporary, and incapacitating pain. Pain persisting longer than 10 minutes suggests more serious urogenital injury. Testicular disease may refer deep, aching pain to the lower abdomen or sacrum.[11,12] The prostate gland refers pain to the lower back, scrotum, or perineum.[11,12]

Female Urogenital System

The uterus refers pain to the middle and lower back, whereas the ovaries and fallopian tubes refer pain to the lower abdomen (suprapubic) and sacrum.[11] Breast pain is usually localized to the affected breast but may refer symptoms to the ipsilateral upper arm.

MEDICAL HISTORY AND PHYSICAL EXAMINATION

Family and Personal History

A history of untreated urinary infection or sexually transmitted disease (see Chapter Nine) can cause significant long-term health problems. A family history of renal disease or personal history of systemic disorders such as diabetes, hypertension, or sickle cell anemia increases risk of urogenital system pathology. Exposure to certain toxins may also affect renal function, including heavy metals, radioactive substances, and medications such as anti-inflammatories, antibiotics, and narcotics.[3]

For young females, age of menarche (first menses) and menstrual history (pain, difficulty, regularity, etc), including date of the last period, should be elicited if a urogenital condition is suggested by their history.[7] Family history of breast cancer, particularly with onset at an early age, is important with complaints of breast pain, mass, or discharge.[13] Both males and females should be asked whether they perform regular self-examinations when presenting symptoms related to the urogenital systems. Sexual dysfunction, urethral discharge, or abnormal menses are symptoms requiring medical referral.

Change in Urinary Habit

Changes in an individual's urinary frequency, particularly if sudden or progressive, can indicate a urogenital disorder. Dysuria (difficult urination), nocturia (frequent waking from sleep to urinate), unusual urgency, and incontinence are symptoms of urogenital pathology. Oliguria (very infrequent urination) and anuria (absence of urination) are results of very serious renal, urinary, or metabolic disorders.

Nipple Discharge

Serous (watery), sanguineous (bloody), or serosanguineous (mixed) discharge may occur with breast cancer and other more benign breast conditions, such as gland infection and hormonal imbalances.[13]

Inspection

Edema in the extremities usually occurs in late-stage kidney disease. Other urogenital conditions present few signs that would be noticeable upon inspection by an athletic trainer.

Palpation

The kidneys, particularly the right kidney, can sometimes be palpated in the posterior thorax near the vertebral column below the costal border of the 12th rib (costovertebral angle). Tenderness upon palpation at this location is abnormal. Pain reproduced by percussion (or "hammering") directly over the kidney indicates inflammation or injury (see Lab Activity 7).[1,14-16]

The athletic trainer relies on history, symptoms, and other signs to raise suspicion of pathology in the genital system. If necessary, the person can be instructed to perform self-examination and report the findings.

Urinalysis

Hematuria (blood in urine), proteinuria (protein in urine), and glucosuria (glucose in urine) can be detected using commercially available urine dipsticks. The chemically treated end of the stick is inserted and removed from a urine sample. Changes on the stick are interpreted according to the indicator or label included with the package of sticks. An abnormal dipstick result requires urgent referral to a physician for more formal medical testing.

In addition, changes in color, odor, or volume of urine may also indicate a urinary disorder. Urine is normally pale yellow but will darken considerably as fluid content decreases or relative concentration of solute increases. Red or brownish urine usually contains blood, hemoglobin, myoglobin, bilirubin, or other metabolic protein and is therefore never normal.[3] A clouded or milky appearance indicates infection, which is usually accompanied by a foul or strong odor.[3] Discolored urine requires appropriate medical urinalysis.

Hypertension

Lab Activity 2 describes the assessment of blood pressure. Chapter Three discusses clinical hypertension.

Anemia

Kidney pathology may affect a hormone that regulates red blood cell production, leading to anemia. Signs and symptoms of anemia are reviewed in Chapter Three.

PATHOLOGY AND PATHOGENESIS

Renal, Bladder, and Genital Trauma

A direct blow to the middle or lower back, sudden deceleration of the trunk, or a fractured rib can injure the kidney. The hallmark of such renal injury is hematuria.[17] Tenderness or swelling may appear over ribs 10 through 12. Grossly observable blood in the urine after a blow to the back or other abdominal trauma requires emergency medical imaging and diagnostic studies. Most kidney trauma can be treated without surgery but demands close medical monitoring. Return to sports is slow, usually taking at least 6 to 8 weeks before evidence of healing by medical imaging is observed.[17] Collision sports are contraindicated for persons who have only a single kidney.

The urethra and bladder may also sustain trauma during physical activity. Significant bladder injuries are rare in athletics and are more common with high-energy injuries, such as a car accident. Hematuria and pain in the lower abdomen usually occur with bladder injuries. More commonly, minor bleeding (exertional hematuria) after long duration or very strenuous activity, such as marathon running, is observed.

Urethral bleeding happens with traumatic impact of the genitals or perineum. If inflammation obstructs the urethra, surgical intervention to allow urine to drain and hospitalization until healed are indicated.[17] The immediate course of action includes application of ice packs and emergency transport.

Renal Disorders

Urolithiasis

Urolithiasis (kidney stone) forms when excess insoluble salts, calcium, or uric acid enter the kidney filtrate. When the stones grow enough to block the flow of urine or irritate the urinary tract, sudden severe pain appears. History is negative for trauma. The characteristic clinical presentation is severe, unilateral pain in the lower back and abdomen that radiates into the anterior thigh.[5] Vomiting, pallor, and tachycardia may also be noted. Signs of shock (decreased BP and rapid, weak pulse) will not be present since no internal hemorrhaging occurs.

Small kidney stones are treated with pain medication and hydration to pass them through the urinary system. Large stones may need to be fragmented by sound, shock, or light (laser). Recovery is usually complete, although recurrences are not uncommon. Risk of kidney stones decreases with properly balanced diet and hydration.[5]

Renal Failure

Acute renal failure occurs as a result of ingested kidney toxins or acute obstruction of the ureter.[5] Signs include sudden weight gain, generalized edema, hypertension, and signs of left-sided heart failure (see Chapter Three).[3]

Chronic renal failure is unlikely among physically active persons. As a complication of diabetes, hypertension, or other kidney disease, however, chronic renal failure is not uncommon among the American population. In early stages, chronic renal failure may be asymptomatic. As the disease progresses, nocturia, hypertension, gastrointestinal symptoms, impaired cognitive function, neurological changes (decreased reflexes, paresthesia), bone degeneration, muscle dysfunction, and cardiovascular complications gradually occur.[2,5] Chronic renal failure is not curable since damaged kidney cells cannot regenerate.

Male Urogenital Disorders

Monorchidism

Monorchidism, or the absence of one testicle, congenitally occurs in .02% (1 in 5000) of males but can be traumatically acquired.[18] This condition often excludes a male from contact sports, as is the unilateral absence of several other paired organs (kidney, eye, etc). More rarely, complete absence of both testicles or the presence of more than two testicles occurs.[18] Decisions regarding sports participation in these conditions should be deferred to a urologist or endocrinologist.

Prostate Disorders

Prostate disorders often gradually produce symptoms that are related to chronic or acute inflammation (prostatitis). The prevalence of prostate disorders increases with age. The most frequent cause of prostatitis is infection, although it can occur with cancer or other urogenital disease.[5] Dysuria, painful urination, an increase in urinary urgency and frequency, and nocturia are commonly reported symptoms.[5,11] In addition, a dull ache may develop in the lower back or sacrum. The gland also enlarges with age (benign prostatic hypertrophy), causing signs and symptoms of chronic prostatitis.[5,11]

Scrotum and Testicular Trauma

The scrotum is vulnerable to trauma in sports, necessitating the use of protective equipment. Unfortunately, male athletes often refuse to use a protective cup consistently. Most scrotum trauma is relatively benign, producing the typical and temporary testicular pain described above. More significant injury can occur, however, such as testicular torsion.[17] Scrotal or testicular pain that does not improve in less than 10 minutes is highly suspicious of a more serious injury.

Testicular Torsion

Testicular torsion occurs primarily during late childhood or adolescence, as the developing scrotum allows rotation of the testis and its connective tissue capsule.[18] The spermatic cord twists, compressing arteries and veins and causing ischemia in the affected testicle.[5]

A history of trauma or previous torsion may be present but is not necessary.[17] Table 6-1 compares benign scrotum trauma with the classic clinical presentation of testicular torsion. Nausea and vomiting are common.[18] The twisted spermatic cord elevates the affected testicle from its normal position. This may be reported by patient report following self-evaluation. Emergency surgery is necessary to save the testicle, even if spontaneous or manual "derotation" occurs.[18]

Varicoceles

Varicose veins in the scrotum (varicoceles) most commonly occur in adolescents and cause a sensation of heaviness or tenderness.[5,18] Varicoceles range in diameter from 1 to 2 cm,

Table 6-1

SIMPLE SCROTUM TRAUMA VS TESTICULAR TORSION

	Scrotum Trauma	Testicular Torsion
Pain	Bilateral, less than 10 minutes	Unilateral, over 10 minutes
Scrotum swelling	None	Progressive
Nausea/vomiting	None or very brief nausea	Increasing nausea and eventual vomiting
Testicular position	Normal	Unilateral elevation

are more prominent when standing, and may be described as a "bag of worms."[18] Surgical correction may be necessary since varicoceles do not spontaneously regress and may lead to fertility problems.[18] Trauma may produce testicular hydrocele, or a fluid-filled sac, which produces similar signs and symptoms to varicocele but with sudden onset after trauma. Medical referral is appropriate.

Female Urogenital Disorders

Endometriosis

Endometriosis occurs when endometrial tissue grows outside the uterus and is most common in women between 30 and 40 years of age.[5,6,11] Menstruation becomes painful and volume of menstrual discharge increases. Painful intercourse and pain in the lower back is also usually reported.[6] Fibrosis and infertility can result, so prompt referral is important. Treatment consists of hormone therapy or surgery.[5]

Pregnancy

Pregnancy, although not a pathological state, does produce signs and symptoms. Pregnancy occurs when a fertilized ovum attaches to the endometrium. Signs and symptoms often appear before the patient knows she is pregnant. Amenorrhea, unexplained weight gain (5 to 10 lbs a month), recurrent nausea and vomiting, and abdominal pain in a female beyond menarche require a physician referral. Other signs and symptoms appear as pregnancy advances, including frequent urination, hypotension in the supine position, peripheral neurovascular occlusion syndromes (from fluid retention and edema), and breast enlargement and tenderness.[6] A weight gain of 25 to 30 lbs during the course of a pregnancy is normal but may cause fatigue and musculoskeletal strain syndromes.[6,19]

Resting heart rate increases early in pregnancy and continues to increase to as much as 15 beats per minute (bpm) over normal throughout the pregnancy.[19] BP, however, progressively decreases, with a change of 8 to 10 mmHg by the 20th week.[6] The decrease in BP is exacerbated in supine during late pregnancy, so exercise in this position should be avoided after the fourth month.[6,19] As a precaution, pregnant women should be taught the symptoms of rapidly decreasing BP, including dizziness, syncope, and nausea so they can change positions to restore BP.[6]

The physician managing prenatal care should be consulted before advising a pregnant woman in any type of exercise program. Conditions such as diabetes, hypertension, history of miscarriage, and presence of multiple fetuses usually render exercise contraindicated.[20] If exercise is recommended, regular, low-impact aerobic exercise (HR below 140 bpm) in 15-minute intervals is usually indicated.[19] Duration and intensity of exercise sessions should be adjusted to avoid elevating body temperature, maternal or fetal injury, exhaustion (ie, depletion of blood glucose), or dehydration.[20] In addition, environment (temperature and safety) and nutrition (additional 300 kcal/day usually recommended throughout pregnancy) should be considered.[19,20]

The circulating concentration of the hormone relaxin increases substantially during pregnancy. Relaxin increases the extensibility of connective tissues, such as ligaments.[6] This renders skeletal joints more susceptible to injury during physical activity and thereby prohibits vigorous sports participation. In addition, precaution is needed during application of manual therapy techniques such as joint mobilization.

Returning to a regular exercise regimen may take several months after delivery. Physical changes of pregnancy often persist up to 6 weeks postpartum (after giving birth).[20] Activities to avoid in the immediate postpartum stage include exercise in hot, humid weather (dehydration), high-impact or high-intensity exercise, excessive stretching or joint motions (due to relaxin), and sudden changes in posture (orthostatic hypotension).[19] An additional 400 to 600 kcal/day may be required for women who are breast-feeding to meet basic metabolic demands.[19]

Ruptured Ectopic Pregnancy

An ectopic pregnancy occurs when a fertilized ovum attaches outside the uterus, usually in a fallopian tube. The usual signs of pregnancy are present after fertilization. When the embryo grows large enough, it ruptures the tube, producing severe internal hemorrhaging. Ruptured ectopic pregnancy presents acute, lacerating lower abdominal pain with lower quadrant tenderness, vaginal bleeding, syncope, and shock.[6,21] Syncope associated with abdominal pain in a female of childbearing age always requires prompt medical attention.[6,21] An embryo implanted ectopically has no chance of surviving. The condition is fatal to the mother unless emergency surgery is performed.[21]

Female Athletic Triad

Female athletic triad describes the simultaneous presence of disordered eating, amenorrhea, and osteoporosis in otherwise healthy young women.[7,8] Each condition can also occur independently, but in this syndrome they are causally related. Restricted caloric intake and abstention from high-fat or high-calorie foods to reduce or maintain body weight are the most common manifestations of disordered eating among athletes (see Chapter Eight). In addition, poor nutrition is also associated with disordered eating.[7]

Athletes with disordered eating have increased pituitary gland activity due to the combined effects of intense exercise and restricted caloric intake, which inhibits hypothalamic hormone release. Pituitary hormone release is then inhibited, resulting in inadequate estrogen and progesterone production from the ovaries, which causes amenorrhea (defined as less than three cycles per year or lack of menstruation for three consecutive months) or oligomenorrhea (three to six menstrual cycles per year, with cycles in excess of 35 days).[7,8]

A low percentage of body fat, once thought to contribute to amenorrhea, is no longer considered a cause. Restricted caloric intake alone induces amenorrhea in athletes who have normal levels of body fat.[7,20] Amenorrhea is caused by an interaction of hormone imbalances and inadequate nutrition, both of which can be consequences of disordered eating.[7,10,20,22] An underlying cause of amenorrhea should always be medically investigated.

Hormone changes and amenorrhea then contribute to development of osteoporosis (inadequate bone formation and premature bone loss).[22] Estrogen inhibits osteoclast activity. When erratic or irregular menstruation causes low estrogen levels, osteoclast activity (resorbing bone) increases and bone density decreases.[7] This is also the mechanism of postmenopausal osteoporosis, common in women over 50 years of age.

Osteoporosis is also observed in young women who have amenorrhea. Osteoporosis (bone loss) among young female athletes can decrease bone mass between 2% and 6% per year. Recovery of bone mass with treatment may not be complete.[7,8] Since 60% to 70% of bone mass is acquired before age 20, adolescent females with osteoporosis may be at increased risk for fractures and other orthopedic complications later in life.[20]

The definitive management of the female athlete triad depends strongly on early recognition. Signs of disordered eating (see Table 9-5) may be detected first. Disordered eating alone has high morbidity (illness) and mortality (death) rates and should be addressed promptly and appropriately (see Chapter Eight). Amenorrhea in athletes, particularly when disordered eating or decreased bone density is detected, requires a decrease in exercise intensity and a change in diet to increase body weight by 2% or 3%, including a daily calcium intake of 1200 to 1500 mg.[8]

Breast Disorders

Breast masses in adult women, changes in breast shape or resiliency, change in size or number of masses, tenderness, or discharge require urgent referral to a physician, particularly if the patient has a positive family history of cancer. In adolescents, however, breast changes and inconsistently tender lumps detected during self-examination are often benign.[13] The proper term for such benign breast changes is *proliferative breast changes*, formerly called *fibrocystic breast disease*.[13] Genetic and hormonal factors are likely, with little to no evidence that caffeine or other lifestyle-related factors contribute.[13] Most cases of proliferative breast changes have no adverse long-term health consequences. Treatment of benign breast lesions is usually observation, aspiration or core biopsy, or surgical excision.[13]

Breast pain may be a result of direct trauma or repetitive strain from activities such as running with poor support.[17] Ice is recommended following a painful blow to the breast. Anti-inflammatories should be avoided since they may increase bleeding and subsequent scarring. Use of a sports bra can prevent repetitive strain injuries.[17]

Ovarian Cysts

Fibrous cysts (vascular, fluid-filled sacs) can form within the female urogenital system, including the ovaries.[5] Although usually asymptomatic and benign, occasionally they cause significant health problems. Ovarian cysts may cause unusual bleeding or interfere with the menstrual cycle.[5] If ovarian cysts are large or numerous (polycystic ovary syndrome), they may interfere with normal estrogen production, causing course hair to grow on the chest and face (hirsutism).[5] Furthermore, ovarian cysts may rupture, producing sudden and severe internal hemorrhaging. Ruptured ovarian cysts lead to abdominal pain, peritonitis, shock, and sometimes death.[5,23,24]

PEDIATRIC CONCERNS

Primary Amenorrhea

Primary amenorrhea is absence of menarche (first menses) by age 16, most commonly caused by hormonal, genetic, or reproductive organ disorders.[20,22] If not already receiving medical care, referral to a pediatrician or gynecologist is appropriate. If uncorrected, primary amenorrhea leads to the problems noted above for other types of amenorrhea.

Kidney Trauma

Among children, kidney injuries are much more frequent than spleen or liver injuries.[17] The kidneys are exposed inferior to the costovertebral angle until adolescence. Hence, a child who has received trauma to the trunk or back should be screened for signs (hematuria, shock) and symptoms (flank pain) of renal damage.

Cryptorchidism

Cryptorchidism, or undescended testes, is the most common congenital abnormality of the male genitalia.[18] Normally, the testes descend from the abdomen into the scrotum just before birth or during the first year of life.[5] Usually detected in infancy during regular pediatric care, cryptorchidism occasionally persists into early childhood. The undescended testes have a high rate of malignancy and infertility if uncorrected (up to 20 times higher than the general male population).[5,18] More important to the athletic trainer is the high rate of inguinal hernia that is associated with cryptorchidism.[18] Although such hernias are usually surgically corrected before the age of 2 years (if detected), a history of cryptorchidism may indicate a recurrent hernia when assessing groin pain.

SUMMARY

The renal-urinary system removes metabolic wastes from the blood and has a major role in regulation of body fluid levels and blood pressure. The signs of renal damage are hematuria, abnormal dipstick test (proteinuria, glucosuria), and hypertension. Symptoms include pain in the back and abdomen, costovertebral angle tenderness, and change in urinary habit (frequency, urgency, volume). The genital or reproductive system contains the organs of procreation specific to each gender. The male genitals are prone to traumatic injury, most of which is temporary and benign. Unilateral scrotum pain or swelling, however, may indicate an emergency condition. The menstrual cycle is an indication of female reproductive system function. If menses is unusually heavy or painful, or very infrequent or absent, pathology may exist in the uterus or ovaries. Pregnancy, while not pathological, produces certain characteristic signs and symptoms and requires precautions both during and after pregnancy to prevent injury to the mother or fetus. The female athletic triad is the simultaneous presence of disordered eating, amenorrhea, and osteoporosis. Early recognition and intervention are necessary to prevent long-term complications. Any sign of renal or genital pathology accompanied by shock indicates internal bleeding and is an emergency.

RESOURCES

Renal-Urogenital

- atlife.com renal (kidney) and urology sites:

  www.atnephrology.com/nephrology

  www.aturology.com/urology

- National Institute of Diabetes and Digestive and Kidney Diseases and National Institutes of Health. www.niddk.nih.gov/health/kidney/kidney.htm

- Yahoo directory. dir.yahoo.com/Health/Diseases_and_Conditions/Kidney_Diseases

REFERENCES

1. Goodman CC, Snyder TEK. Overview of renal and urologic signs and symptoms. In: Goodman CC, Snyder TEK, eds. *Differential Diagnosis in Physical Therapy: Musculoskeletal and Systemic Conditions*. 3rd ed. Philadelphia, Pa: WB Saunders Company; 2000:234-259.

2. McLinn DM, Boissonnault WG. Screening for male urogenital system disease. In: Boissonnault WG, ed. *Examination in Physical Therapy Practice: Screening for Medical Disease*. 2nd ed. New York: Churchill Livingstone Inc; 1995:117-132.

3. Andreoli TE, Culpepper RM, Thompson CS, et al. Section III-renal disease. In: Andreoli TE, Carpenter CCJ, Plum F, et al, eds. *Cecil's Essentials of Medicine*. 2nd ed. Philadelphia, Pa: WB Saunders Company; 1990:176-252.

4. Ganong WF. *Review of Medical Physiology*. 15th ed. Norwalk, Conn: Appleton & Lange; 1991.

5. Gould BE. Urinary system disorders. *Pathophysiology for the Health-Related Professions*. Philadelphia, Pa: WB Saunders Company; 1997:299-319.

6. King PM, Ling FW, Myers CA. Screening for female urogenital system disease. In: Boissonnault WG, ed. *Examination in Physical Therapy Practice: Screening for Medical Disease*. 2nd ed. New York: Churchill Livingstone Inc; 1995:133-153.

7. Putukian M. The female athlete triad. *Clin Sports Med*. 1998;17(4):675-696.

8. West RV. The female athlete: the triad of disordered eating, amenorrhea, and osteoporosis. *Sports Med*. 1998;26(2):63-71.

9. Abarbanel J, Benet AE, Lask D, et al. Sports hematuria. *J Urol*. 1990;143:887-890.

10. Wilson CA, Abdenour TE, Keye WR. Menstrual disorders among intercollegiate athletes and non-athletes: perceived impact on performance, preventative medical care for the female athlete. *Athletic Training*. 1991;26(2):170-177.

11. Boissonnault WG, Bass C. Pathological origins of trunk and neck pain, part I: pelvic and abdominal visceral disorders. *J Orthop Sports Phys Ther*. 1990;12(5):192-207.

12. Stopka CB, Zambito KL. Referred visceral pain: what every sports medicine professional needs to know. *Athletic Therapy Today*. 1999;4(1):29-36.

13. Neinstein LS. Breast disease in adolescents and young women. *Pediatr Clin North Am*. 1999;46(3):607-629.

14. Bickley LS, Hoekelman RA. *Bates' Guide to Physical Examination and History Taking*. 7th ed. Philadelphia, Pa: Lippincott Williams & Wilkins; 1999.

15. Boissonnault WG, ed. *Examination in Physical Therapy Practice: Screening for Medical Disease*. 2nd ed. New York: Churchill Livingstone; 1995.

16. DeGowin RL, Brown DD. *DeGowin's Diagnostic Examination.* 7th ed. New York: McGraw-Hill; 2000.

17. Amaral JF. Thoracoabdominal injuries in the athlete. *Clin Sports Med.* 1997;16(4):739-753.

18. Pillai SB, Besner GE. Pediatric testicular problems. *Pediatr Clin North Am.* 1998;45(4):813-830.

19. Artal R. Exercise and pregnancy. *Clin Sports Med.* 1992;11(2):363-377.

20. Teitz CC, Hu SS, Arendt EA. The female athlete: evaluation and treatment of sports-related problems. *J Am Acad Orthop Surg.* 1997;5(2):87-96.

21. Stone R. Primary care diagnosis of acute abdominal pain. *Nurse Practitioner.* 1996;21(12):19-20, 23-26, 28-30, 35-41.

22. Worthington G. Athletic amenorrhea: updated review. *Athletic Training.* 1991;26(3):270-273.

23. Giudice L. Menstrual abnormalities and abnormal uterine bleeding. In: Beers MH, Berkow R, eds. *The Merck Manual of Diagnosis and Therapy.* 17th ed. Whitehouse Station, NJ: Merck Research Laboratories; 1999:1932-1942.

24. Hendrix S. Pelvic pain. In: Beers MH, Berkow R, eds. *The Merck Manual of Diagnosis and Therapy.* 17th ed. Whitehouse Station, NJ: Merck Research Laboratories; 1999:1944-1948.

Chapter Seven

Endocrine and Metabolic Systems

PURPOSES

- Describe the basic endocrine system structures and their functions.
- Review pathophysiological mechanisms of the endocrine system, including contributions to homeostasis and metabolism.
- Describe the response of the endocrine system to exercise.
- Describe basic metabolic responses to exercise.
- Discuss medical history findings relevant to endocrine and metabolic pathology.
- Identify signs and symptoms of endocrine pathology.
- Identify signs and symptoms of metabolic pathology.
- Perform physical examination tasks relevant to the endocrine system and normal metabolism.
- Discuss, compare, and contrast selected endocrine pathology and metabolic disorders.

Figure 7-1. Glands of the endocrine system.

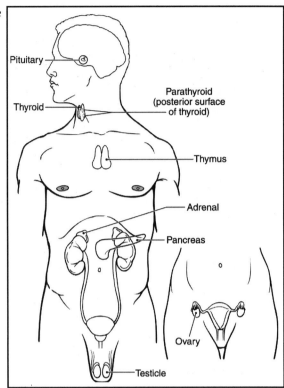

INTRODUCTION

The endocrine system consists of several glands throughout the body (Figure 7-1). Hormones are complex proteins secreted by the endocrine glands into the blood to produce various actions in the organ systems of the body, including inhibition or stimulation of other hormones. Table 7-1 lists the endocrine glands and their primary hormones.[1,2] The endocrine system receives input from the nervous, gastrointestinal, cardiovascular, hepatic, and renal systems. Actions of the hormones regulate the internal environment and function of the body, thus contributing substantially to homeostasis.

Metabolism describes the biochemical functions and interaction of the organ systems of the body. These processes respond to the normal cyclic increases and decreases in organ activity, internal energy demands, environmental factors, and nutrition. Metabolic activity is regulated internally by hormones and organs but also by external physical factors and intake of calories, carbohydrates, protein, fat, water, minerals, and vitamins. Thus, metabolism is the manifestation of the endocrine system's attempt to maintain homeostasis.

Table 7-1

ENDOCRINE GLANDS, SELECTED ASSOCIATED HORMONES, AND HORMONE FUNCTIONS

Gland	Hormone(s)	Hormone Function
Pituitary-hypothalamus	Growth hormone	Increases protein synthesis
Pituitary	Adrenocorticotropic hormone	Causes adrenals to release cortisol
	Thyroid-stimulating hormone	Increases thyroid function
	Follicle-stimulating hormone	Increases estrogen release (females) Increases sperm production (males)
	Luteinizing hormone	Stimulates ovulation (females) Increases testosterone release (males)
	Antidiuretic hormone	Increases water absorption in the kidneys
Thyroid	Thyroid hormone	Increases metabolism
	Calcitonin	Decreases demineralization of bone
Parathyroid	Parathyroid hormone	Increases calcium in the blood by demineralizing bone
Adrenal	Aldosterone	Increases water absorption in kidneys
	Cortisol	Anti-inflammatory, tissue catabolism, responds to stress
	Epinephrine	Responds to stress (increase heart rate, increase blood flow to muscle, decrease blood flow to internal organs)
	Norepinephrine	Vasoconstriction
Pancreas (endocrine)	Insulin	Increases glucose transport out of blood and into cells
	Glucagon	Releases glucose from the liver into blood
Testes	Testosterone	Produces secondary male sex characteristics, increases protein synthesis, increases sperm production, inhibits luteinizing hormone release
Ovaries	Estrogen	Produces secondary female sex characteristics, regulates menstrual cycle, inhibits luteinizing hormone release
	Progesterone	Produces secondary female sex characteristics, regulates menstrual cycle, inhibits estrogen activity

REVIEW OF ANATOMY, PHYSIOLOGY, AND PATHOGENESIS

Regulation of Body Energy

Carbohydrate (glucose) in the blood is the body's primary energy source. A system of hormones regulates blood carbohydrate level (normally about 10 mg/dL), including insulin and glucagon from the pancreas, epinephrine and norepinephrine from the adrenals, and growth hormone from the pituitary gland. All of these hormones except insulin release glucose from glycogen stores, increasing carbohydrates available for use by the body. Conversely, as blood carbohydrate level increases after eating, insulin removes glucose from the blood and stores it as glycogen in the liver and muscles. During exercise, insulin decreases as metabolic glucose demand increases. Glucose is released in response to this increased fuel demand, primarily through the function of glucagon.[3,4] Simultaneously, insulin receptors on muscle cells become hypersensitive to increase the muscular uptake of glucose, allowing a relative increase in muscle glucose without significant changes in blood insulin level.[3] Epinephrine and norepinephrine (and growth hormone and cortisol during extended exercise) inhibit insulin production, thereby aiding the release of glucose from the liver.[3]

Regulation of Body Temperature

Normal metabolic processes produce excess energy at rest. Most of this energy is released as heat, which maintains the body's temperature within a narrow range. The body can also regulate heat loss or heat production in response to environmental conditions.[5] The hypothalamus, which is sensitive to blood temperature, increases or decreases thyroid-stimulating hormone in the pituitary gland. In response to decreases in body temperature, increased thyroid-stimulating hormone increases thyroid hormone, which causes metabolism to increase. Higher metabolism requires more energy-producing biochemical reactions, which then increases body temperature. Through opposite reactions, increased body temperature decreases thyroid-stimulating hormone and thus lowers metabolism and consequently inhibits body temperature from further increasing.

With initiation of exercise, core body temperature rises slightly and the physiological heat-dissipating mechanisms begin to function, primarily evaporation of water from the skin (ie, sweating) and radiation of heat from the head and neck. Ideally, a steady state is reached in which heat production and heat dissipation stabilizes body temperature.[5]

Regulation of Body Fluid Levels

Antidiuretic hormone (ADH) forms in the hypothalamus and is secreted by the pituitary gland.[6] ADH retains water in the body by facilitating water reabsorption from the kidneys, thus decreasing urine volume. Exercise increases ADH secretion when baroreceptors (sensitive to pressure) detect a decrease in blood volume and the hypothalamus detects an increase in blood solutes.[7] Maintaining hydration during activity inhibits this mechanism from secreting ADH since, when properly hydrated, there is no need to retain water.

Hormonal Response To Exercise

Exercise, or any other physical stress, causes a release of hypothalamic, pituitary, and adrenal hormones. As an adaptation to chronic exercise, these reactions decrease with successively higher levels of conditioning. Relatively intense exercise also stimulates release of growth hormone, which increases with higher levels of fitness. Intensity of exercise appears to be the most important factor for growth hormone release. Endurance exercise, however, increases the level of cortisol, which decreases growth hormone secretion. Thus, a potential effect of overtraining is a net decrease in growth hormone. Adverse effects, such as stunted height and physical development problems, can occur with combined overtraining and nutritional deficiencies among young female athletes. Secretion of catecholamines (epinephrine and norepinephrine) occurs with onset of exercise but does not appear to adapt with conditioning.

Very frequently, intense exercise depresses follicle-stimulating hormone and lutenizing hormone and, subsequently, decreases secretion of estrogen and (to a lesser extent) testosterone. Decreased estrogen can produce primary amenorrhea among young female athletes but usually only when excessive exercise is accompanied by nutritional deficiency (see Chapter Six). Although circulating testosterone also decreases with endurance exercise, delay of male puberty is very rare, possibly because a much higher exercise intensity is needed in males to depress testosterone release through this mechanism. Occasionally, highly active males report depressed libido (psychoemotional sex drive) and decreased semen volume, although these effects may be caused by dehydration, immune system depression, or undetected systemic illness rather than exercise-induced hormone changes.

Neurotransmitters known as endorphins, or endogenous opiates, are released during exercise of moderate to high intensity. Endorphins are thought to have a mild analgesic effect and counteract cortisol (which is also released during exercise). Additionally, endorphins stimulate lipolysis (breakdown of stored fat) to provide carbohydrates to working muscles.

SIGNS AND SYMPTOMS

Skin Changes

Some endocrine disorders produce changes in the color, texture, or appearance of the skin. Hormones control melanin (skin pigment) activity and can thus affect skin pigmentation. Changes in skin thickness, flexibility, texture, and strength may appear in response to pathological conditions of the endocrine system.

Hyperhydrosis/Diaphoresis and Body/Breath Odor

Diaphoresis (sweating) or *hyperhydrosis* (excessive sweating) occurs if metabolism increases. Diaphoresis is a normal response to exercise. Metabolic imbalance or endocrine disorders, however, can cause hyperhydrosis at rest. Elevated body temperature or release of catecholamines (epinephrine and norepinephrine) can also cause profuse sweating.

High blood glucose produces a very sweet odor on the breath and body. Metabolic breakdown of toxins and other organic substances can be exhaled or secreted in breath, sweat, and urine, where they can be detected by smell (eg, alcohol, drugs).

Polydipsia and Polyuria

Excessive thirst (polydipsia) or urination (polyuria) can be caused by inadequate secretion of ADH or thyroid disorders.[6]

Arthralgia and Myalgia

Joint (arthralgia) and muscle (myalgia) pain are common with the disturbance of endocrine function or metabolism. Multiple joints or muscles are usually involved and the pattern is bilateral and symmetric.

Muscle Atrophy and Weakness

Changes in muscle function and structure are results of insufficient nutrition (either starvation or as a result of disease) or the chronic presence of catabolic hormones (eg, cortisol, epinephrine). Many endocrine disorders also affect muscle energy metabolism, causing unusual weakness and atrophy.

Amenorrhea and Impotence

Function of the reproductive organs and mechanisms can be affected by disorders involving the hypothalamus, pituitary gland, ovaries, or testes.

Confusion or Change in Mental Status

Cognitive function can be affected by many endocrine-metabolic disorders, including hypoglycemia, dehydration, abnormal body temperature, or insufficient nutrition.

Paresthesia

Long-term endocrine or metabolic disorders can cause damage to nerve cells, axons, or myelin, causing progressive peripheral paresthesia.

Edema and Pitting Edema

Extracellular fluid can accumulate with certain endocrine or metabolic system disorders.

Polyphagia

Excessive intake of food suggests overactive thyroid production, nutritional deficits, or metabolic imbalances.

Postural (Orthostatic) Hypotension

The endocrine system regulates fluid levels in the blood. If blood volume decreases (through excessive urination or dehydration), blood pressure decreases rapidly with a change in posture from lying or sitting to standing.

Lethargy and Fatigue

Since the endocrine system regulates metabolism, disorders in this system affect availability and utilization of oxygen and energy. Fatigue and lethargy (abnormal sluggishness, drowsiness, or indifference) result either from an overactive metabolism requiring large energy expenditures or from an underactive metabolism depriving the body of energy. In addition, many endocrine conditions directly or indirectly (eg, through nocturia) affect sleep quality and duration, leading to fatigue from sleep deprivation.

PAIN PATTERNS

The endocrine glands rarely produce pain directly. The signs and symptoms of hormonal imbalances are usually more relevant than reports of pain.

Hypothalamus and Pituitary

Large tumors in these glands can produce headache or visual disturbances by compressing the brain.

Thyroid and Parathyroid

Tenderness in the anterior, inferior aspect of the throat and neck may be palpated or produced during extension of the head (stretching the anterior neck).

Adrenals

Adrenal disorders produce widespread myalgia and arthralgia (see Table 7-1).

Pancreas

The pancreas produces upper left quadrant or generalized epigastric pain, as discussed in Chapter Five under *Pain Patterns*. Extensive pancreatic disease is required before pain is produced.

MEDICAL HISTORY AND PHYSICAL EXAMINATION

Family and Personal History

Certain metabolic disorders, such as diabetes mellitus, have a very strong genetic component that may be evident in a family history. Metabolic disturbances can also be caused by environmental factors (eg, temperature, toxins, physical stress), so these should be investigated during the medical history. Many endocrine disorders produce a characteristic pattern or progression of symptoms that can be detected through a careful medical history.

Physical Examination

Skin appearance and characteristics, secondary sex characteristics, muscle atrophy, unusual hair patterns in females, hyperhydrosis, odor of breath or perspiration, edema, postural hypotension, and paresthesia may all be related to endocrine system disorders. Observation and testing vital signs (particularly heart rate and blood pressure) may be the only physical tests used to detect potential endocrine pathology. An enlarged thyroid can be both seen and palpated lateral to the trachea above the clavicles.[8] An abnormally enlarged thyroid (goiter) is a sign of thyroid toxicity, iodine deficiency, or thyroid pathology. Most endocrine diseases require medical laboratory testing to confirm the diagnosis.

PATHOLOGY AND PATHOGENESIS

Diabetes Mellitus

Insulin-Dependent Diabetes Mellitus (Type I)

Type I diabetes mellitus, or insulin-dependent diabetes mellitus (IDDM), affects approximately one in 500 children and adolescents.[3,4] An autoimmune disease, IDDM destroys the insulin-producing cells of the endocrine pancreas.[9] Without insulin, the body cannot regulate blood glucose level. Persons with IDDM require insulin injections several times daily to facilitate glucose uptake by muscles and the liver. IDDM has no cure. The person must maintain a strict, lifelong medical and dietary regimen to control carbohydrate metabolism. Long-term health consequences of IDDM include peripheral and autonomic neuropathy, retinopathy (blindness), cardiovascular disease, hypertension, kidney disorders, chronic skin ulcers, and poor healing capability.[9] Persons with poorly controlled glucose levels have a higher risk of severe complications.[10] Regular aerobic exercise indirectly inhibits the development or advancement of some complications among people with IDDM.

Generally, significant health problems do not occur for at least 10 years after the onset of disease in patients with good control. Risk of complications increases with age. Children and adolescents who maintain a good insulin and diet program can participate in most sports with few or no precautions. Adults with poorly controlled IDDM are at substantial risk for cardiovascular pathology and should exercise only under medical advice and guidelines.[11]

The athletic trainer should be aware of the signs of hypo- and hyperglycemia (Table 7-2) and be prepared to handle these emergencies in persons with IDDM.[12] Hypoglycemia occurs during physical exertion with a high level of circulating insulin, usually after an insulin injection and failure to eat before exercising.[11,12] Hyperglycemia, conversely, occurs with an excessive release of glucose in response to exercise, most likely when glucose level is already very high (> 220 mg/dl) before exercise begins.[10,11]

Since exercise affects glucose levels, athletes with IDDM should discuss adjustment of insulin type, dose, or regimen with their physician.[10,11] In addition, persons with IDDM may have a significant hypoglycemic response 6 to 24 hours after strenuous exercise.[3,4,11,12] A post-exercise insulin dose may need to be decreased and the post-exercise meal should ensure adequate caloric intake.[4] Conversely, failure to inject insulin after exercise causes hyperglycemia since glucose released during exercise is not countered by insulin secretion. Competitive athletes need to adhere to specific regimens to maintain blood glucose control, including injection schedules, frequent blood glucose monitoring, and strict diet.[4,9-11]

Table 7-2

SIGNS OF HYPERGLYCEMIA AND HYPOGLYCEMIA IN A PERSON WITH DIABETES MELLITUS

Hyperglycemia: diabetic ketoacidosis, diabetic coma, or diabetic hyperosmolar state

- Blood glucose over 300 mg/dl
- Gradual onset
- Abdominal pain
- Thirst but not hunger
- Fruity odor on the breath (acetone)

- Dehydration
- Lethargy
- Confusion
- Loss of consciousness (coma)

Hypoglycemia: insulin shock

- Blood glucose below 70 mg/dl
- Sudden onset
- Headache
- Hunger but not thirst
- Blurred vision
- Dizziness

- Decreased performance
- Autonomic signs (pallor, diaphoresis, tachycardia, tremors)
- Fatigue
- Slurred speech
- Confusion

Noninsulin-Dependent Diabetes Mellitus (Type II)

Type II diabetes mellitus, or noninsulin-dependent diabetes mellitus (NIDDM), is a disorder characterized by normal or high levels of insulin but decreased insulin receptor sensitivity. Thus, glucose uptake by the liver and muscles is substantially impaired.[3,4] Until recently, NIDDM was primarily a disease of adults, but the disorder has been gradually increasing among children. NIDDM affects 10 to 20 million people in the United States, many of whom are unaware they have the condition.[4,8]

Chronically elevated blood glucose level eventually produces hyperlipidemia (elevated fat level in blood), arteriosclerosis (hardening of the arteries), peripheral neuropathy, chronic infections, and bone changes (eg, osteoporosis).[8] A positive family history of NIDDM and obesity are strong predictors of this condition.[4] Polydipsia and polyuria are the most common symptoms of NIDDM.[8] Increased fluid intake (polydipsia) occurs to dilute blood glucose concentration but causes an increase in excretion by the kidneys (polyuria).

Low-to-moderate intensity exercise facilitates muscle glucose uptake among persons with NIDDM.[10,13] Exercise and a controlled diet are mainstays in the prevention and treatment of NIDDM.[4,10] Exercise directly affects blood glucose level by increasing the metabolic demand of muscle and increasing the effectiveness of insulin receptors. The risk of hypoglycemia during exercise for persons with NIDDM is very low (since it only occurs after insulin injection).[4]

Generally speaking, adolescents who have either type of diabetes have no particular precautions to any activity if glucose levels are well controlled.[4,10] Aerobic exercise, however, has certain advantages for persons with diabetes: does not increase blood pressure (which would increase the risk of retinopathy or nephropathy); decreases potential for skin wounds; assists in increasing insulin receptor sensitivity; produces cardiovascular benefits (eg, lowering blood lipids); and provides weight control (particularly for NIDDM).[3,10]

Table 7-3

MANAGING THE ATHLETE WITH DIABETES MELLITUS

1. Obtain frequency of hypoglycemia episodes in the preparticipation examination.
2. Communicate with the doctor relative to adjusting insulin dose and schedule specific to the type of exercise.
3. Take blood glucose reading before practice or competition and take appropriate action:
   - <100 mg/dl = carbohydrate snack before practice
   - >250 mg/dl = no practice, urinalysis for ketones (energy), and insulin injection
4. Communicate with the athlete and coach to leave practice immediately at the first sign of hypoglycemia.
5. Have a ready source of simple carbohydrate (eg, hard candy, fruit juice) available at all times.
6. Establish an emergency plan for severe hypoglycemia with the athlete and the athlete's physician or team physician, including injecting glucagon or intravenous glucose if available.

During the preparticipation examination of a person with diabetes, reports of frequent previous hypoglycemic episodes suggest poor glucose control.[4] Preparticipation meals should be adjusted for both expected exercise intensity and blood glucose level at the time of the meal.[11] Approximately 15 to 30 grams of carbohydrate per half hour of athletic exercise may be needed to prevent hypoglycemia.[4,9] A plan for insulin and glucagon availability and administration in the event of hyperglycemia should be established between the athlete, athlete's parents, athletic trainer, and physician.[9]

Immediately before exercise, a blood glucose level below 100 mg/dl necessitates a carbohydrate snack to raise blood glucose. A reading over 250 mg/dl should prohibit exercise and requires urinalysis for ketones, which are metabolic byproducts of fat metabolism (since fat is used as a primary energy source when glucose is unavailable). If ketones are present (a sign of impending diabetic ketoacidosis), insulin is administered, and the person is transported for medical examination and monitoring.[4,9,12] A source of quick glucose (eg, fruit juice, hard candy, etc) should be available during practice and competition to counteract acute hypoglycemia.[4,9,10,12] Table 7-3 outlines the management of athletes with diabetes mellitus.

Additional potential risks for athletes with diabetes are orthostatic hypotension and increased risk for dehydration, both consequences of polyuria decreasing blood volume.[4,12] With awareness and simple precautions, most athletes with diabetes mellitus can participate in sports without restriction or complications.[4,11]

Disorders of the Pituitary Gland

Diabetes Insipidus

Inadequate secretion of ADH from the pituitary gland causes diabetes insipidus.[6] Decreased ADH level prevents water from being reabsorbed in the kidneys, thus producing large amounts of dilute urine.[6] Polyuria and polydipsia with normal blood glucose levels characterize this disorder. Most cases are idiopathic (no discernable cause) but can be caused by tumors, infection, or vascular problems that affect the hypothalamus or pituitary gland.[6]

Acromegaly

Overproduction of growth hormone causes a condition called acromegaly.[8] Excess growth hormone causes continual growth of bones and soft tissues. Persons with acromegaly are usually tall, have a thick prominent jaw (mandible), protruding frontal bone (forehead), large thick hands and feet, a "barrel" chest, and thoracic kyphosis.[8] Some organ systems, including cardiovascular, renal, and digestive, are affected by both the excess growth hormone and the metabolic stress of maintaining a large, continually growing body. Abuse of human growth hormone as an ergogenic aid can produce similar physical characteristics and clinical syndromes.

Disorders of the Thyroid and Parathyroid

Hyperthyroidism

An excess of thyroid hormone impairs glucose metabolism such that muscle has difficulty maintaining exercise.[14] In addition, core body temperature increases abnormally at rest and with exercise. Monitoring for signs of hyperthermia during exercise is warranted.[14,15] Heart rate response to exercise may be greater than normal.[15]

Graves' disease is the most common form of hyperthyroidism, identified by tremors, weakness, difficulty swallowing or speaking, fatigue, and facial or eye motor disorders (tics).[6,8] Hyperthyroidism is treated with medication, radiation, or surgery to inhibit or remove the thyroid gland, depending on the severity and stage of disease.

Hypothyroidism

Inadequate thyroid hormone decreases cardiac output by both limiting heart rate (bradycardia) and left ventricle contractility.[14] Furthermore, the normal peripheral vasodilatation during exercise may not occur. The net effect is decreased oxygen and glucose available to exercising muscle, thus limiting endurance.[14] Signs and symptoms of hypothyroidism include dry skin, weakness, myalgia, bilateral paresthesia, peripheral nonpitting edema, bradycardia, and poor peripheral circulation.[6,8] Thyroid hormone replacement is the usual course of treatment. Although exercise is not contraindicated, muscle damage may occur with relatively little exertion.[15]

Parathyroid Hormone Disorders

Hyperparathyroidism and hypoparathyroidism, or excess or inadequate secretion of parathyroid hormone (respectively), are rarely encountered in athletes. Parathyroid hormone regulates calcium metabolism. Hyperparathyroidism causes excess calcium release (primarily from bone) into the bloodstream. The most obvious consequences are muscle weakness, arthralgia in the hands and feet, and hyperactive reflexes.[6] If untreated, kidney stones, peptic ulcers, and cognitive changes occur.[8] Hypoparathyroidism, conversely, creates a deficiency of blood calcium, leading to muscle spasms during activity, cardiac arrhythmia, thin hair, and brittle nails.[6] Hyper- and hypoparathyroidism also cause symptoms in the gastrointestinal, neurological, and urogenital systems. Surgical removal of the glands is the treatment of hyperparathyroidism, whereas calcium and vitamin D supplements are used for hypoparathyroidism.[8]

Disorders of the Adrenals

Addison's Disease

Addison's disease is inadequate secretion of the adrenal hormones (aldosterone and cortisol). Hyperpigmentation (bronzing) of the skin, fatigue, hypotension, weakness, gastrointestinal (GI) symptoms, and joint pain are common.[6] Fluid and electrolyte imbalances from decreased aldosterone cause dehydration and impaired cardiac output.[15] Tolerance for physical or emotional stress decreases, coordination declines, and hypoglycemia may occur between meals.[15] If untreated, Addison's disease is fatal. Lifetime pharmacological corticosteroids are usually prescribed as treatment. Fluid and electrolyte levels should be maintained, particularly during exercise. The side effects of long-term corticosteroid therapy (see Cushing's syndrome) become more prominent with age. Persons with Addison's disease should have ready access to hydrocortisone to counteract acute adrenal crisis, which exhibits signs of shock and hypoglycemia.[15]

Cushing's Syndrome

Cushing's syndrome is an overproduction of aldosterone and cortisol, producing classic signs of "moon face," pendulous abdomen with stretch marks (sometimes called "central obesity"), muscle atrophy, easy and frequent bruising, and impaired wound healing. Cortisol acts as a very potent anti-inflammatory and often inhibits the signs of infection or tissue damage. In addition, emotional disturbances, decreased libido, NIDDM (from depression of insulin receptors), and masculinization in females (increased body and facial hair, deepened voice, and breast atrophy) eventually occur.[6,8] Surgery, radiation, and adrenal suppression medication are the courses of treatment.[8]

Chronic corticosteroid use produces a similar syndrome, increasing risk for tissue injury during strenuous activity. Electrolyte imbalances, hypertension, and edema are also common. Athletic trainers may encounter patients with chronic inflammatory disorders (arthritis, asthma, etc) who regularly take prescribed corticosteroids as treatment.

Thermoregulation and Environmental Conditions

Thermoregulatory mechanisms are less effective in very young and very old persons. In addition, nutrition, drugs and alcohol, and fitness level affect the ability of the body to disperse or retain heat.[5,16] Persons with seizure disorders or sickle cell anemia may also be predisposed to conditions caused by thermoregulatory disorders.[16]

During exercise in hot environments, large amounts of sweat are produced to cool the body by evaporation. Simultaneously, peripheral vasodilatation supplies muscles with additional oxygen and glucose and provides an increased surface area for heat to dissipate through the skin. These mechanisms create a relative hypovolemia, which decreases stroke volume (see Chapter Three). As a result, heart rate increases to maintain cardiac output.

If hypovolemia continues to increase from dehydration, vasoconstriction occurs in the periphery, thus impairing heat dissipation mechanisms. Central (core) body temperature rises as a consequence. If hydration is not restored, the process progresses, heart rate increases, cardiac output decreases, and blood pressure decreases, eventually producing shock.[17] Several stages of this pathological process, called heat illness (heat cramps, heat exhaustion, and heat stroke), theoretically exist.

Heat Cramps

Heat cramps occur in leg and trunk muscles during exercise in hot weather after mild dehydration.[18] Athletes who are accustomed to exercise in heat (acclimatized) produce very dilute sweat, which preserves salt. Unacclimatized athletes, however, secrete a relatively high concentration of salt in their sweat. Attempts to replace fluid loss with plain water may further dilute the blood and cause muscle spasms from decreased electrolyte (sodium and potassium) levels.[5]

Gradual acclimatization is usually preventative. During an attack of heat cramps, cooling, rehydration, and a dilute (0.1% to 1.0%) saline solution can be used.[18] Once an athlete has experienced heat cramps, a couple days of rest from practice and a gradual return is indicated. Increased dietary salt intake is not necessary and may actually contribute to heat cramps by stimulating sweat glands to secrete even more salt.[5]

Heat Exhaustion

Advanced dehydration, usually from failure to adequately replace lost fluid or electrolytes, produces heat exhaustion.[16,18] The signs and symptoms, although variable, include profuse sweating, rising body temperature (100° to 106°F), tachycardia, hyperpnea, hypotension, headache, fatigue, and nausea.[5,16,18] Changes in mental status are usually not present, although the athlete may physically collapse.[5]

Rapid cooling with cool towels, a cool shower, rest in air conditioning, and rehydration with a very dilute electrolyte drink (0.1% saline content) usually precipitate recovery.[5] Rehydration with large amounts of plain water may dilute the blood, thus accentuating electrolyte depletion.[16] Avoiding extreme heat, acclimatization, and proper rehydration during exercise can prevent heat exhaustion.

Heat Stroke

Heat stroke, a medical emergency with a very high rate of mortality, occurs with body temperatures over 107.5°F (hyperthermia). It is the third leading cause of sport-related death, after head and neck trauma and cardiac failure.[16] Severe dehydration and hypovolemia inhibit the sweating mechanism, which causes the peripheral vascular system to collapse in an attempt to preserve blood pressure to the vital organs.[5] When this occurs, the body cannot dissipate heat and central body temperature increases very quickly. Cardiac output eventually falls so low it cannot maintain blood flow to the brain and kidneys, which produces a reflex-systemic vasodilatation. Vasodilatation greatly increases cardiac demand in an insufficient cardiovascular system, which results in heart failure. Loss of consciousness, convulsions, coma, and death result.[5]

An athlete exercising in a hot environment who has tachycardia, very high body temperature (often palpated or felt radiating from the body), incoordination, physical collapse, and altered cognitive ability (ie, disorientation, confusion, seizure, or hallucination) suggests heat stroke. Drastic emergency measures should be undertaken immediately. Rapid cooling by immersion, showering, or cold towels during immediate transport to a medical emergency room are indicated.[5,18] Intravenous fluids need to be administered under medical direction since hyperhydration can cause pulmonary or cerebral edema.

Deaths during athletic events that are attributable to environmental heat are preventable, in contrast to most cardiac incidents and head injuries. First, a period of acclimatization should be allowed, during which the cardiovascular system and sweating mechanism can adapt.[5,18] Usually physiological acclimatization begins within several days but takes weeks to become effective.[16] Second, and most obvious, vigorous exercise during the hottest part of the day should be avoided or drills and practice moved indoors whenever feasible. For over 50 years, sports medicine practitioners have been issuing guidelines for exercise in hot, humid conditions. Most of these recommendations are unheeded since they effectively prohibit exercise for large portions of outdoor sports seasons in the southern United States.[19] Third, appropriate clothing, avoidance of diuretics such as alcohol and caffeine, and continuous monitoring of athletes during practice can prevent many heat illnesses.[5]

Last, proper rehydration maintains thermoregulatory and cardiovascular function. Fluid loss during intense exercise exceeds the capability to take in water, thus producing dehydration in proportion to exercise duration.[5,17] During shorter, less intense events (up to 1 hour), plain water can be used to rehydrate.[18] Replacement of electrolytes and to some extent carbohydrates in addition to water becomes more important as intensity and duration of exercise increases.[5,17] During endurance events and in between practices, however, plain water increases urine output even when mildly dehydrated. Thus, a carbohydrate-electrolyte drink (solute content between 3% and 6% will not slow gastric emptying and is absorbed in the intestine just as readily as water) may be preferred.[17] An athlete who has lost 3% or more of his or her body weight during exercise in heat should be held from subsequent practices until body weight is restored.

Exposure to Cold

Prolonged exposure to cold environmental temperatures can also cause medical problems, some of which are life-threatening, particularly if moisture and wind are also present. Water has 25 times the heat conductance of air, so wet clothes, rain or sleet, or immersion in cold water quickly removes body heat through conduction.[5] Wind chill, the effect of convection on the skin, can also substantially reduce body temperature, which is compounded if running or moving against the wind.[5,18] In addition, at least half of the body's expelled heat radiates through the head and neck during exercise. Appropriate clothing or protective gear should protect against rain, snow, and wind, as well as adequately cover the head and neck to prevent excessive heat loss.

Frostbite

Frostbite, although rarely fatal, can cause severe tissue damage or limb loss.[20] As exposed skin temperature decreases, a transient blanching and paresthesia called frostnip occurs.[20] This condition is quickly reversible with rewarming (moving indoors) and protecting the area from further exposure.[20]

With prolonged exposure, superficial frostbite, which is limited to the upper layers of the skin, occurs as ice crystals form in extracellular spaces.[20] The skin appears waxy, dry, or cyanotic, and becomes hardened over the joints.[5,18] Ice in the tissues draws fluid from the cells, causing permanent damage to epithelial cells and blood vessels.[20] Once blood supply is disrupted, hypoxic necrosis occurs unless blood can be delivered through adjacent vessels. This tissue hypoxia is the primary cause of tissue damage in frostbite.[16]

Continued exposure progresses to deep frostbite, which involves the deep layers of skin and possibly muscle or other underlying tissues.[18,20] The mechanism of tissue damage is the same as superficial frostbite: ice formation and hypoxia from vascular destruction. The appearance of cyanosis, blood blisters, or completely frozen skin indicates extensive, irreversible tissue damage.[16]

Once frostbite is recognized, prompt removal from the cold should be undertaken. Weightbearing, pressure, or friction of the frostbitten area should be avoided. Wet clothing can be removed if it is not frozen to the skin and replaced with dry, soft blankets or other cloth. The area should not be thawed if refreezing is a possibility, since refreezing increases the extent of tissue damage. Rapid rewarming of the frostbitten limb can be performed by warm water (104° to 108°F, 40° to 42°C) immersion.[5,20] During rewarming, intense pain, bright erythema, edema, and eventually blistering occur as blood supply returns.[5] With large regions of frostbite, transport to a medical facility is required since compartment syndromes and infection are common.

Hypothermia

Prolonged exposure to cold environmental temperatures can produce a potentially serious condition called hypothermia, a central body temperature below 94°F (34.4°C).[20] As central body temperature decreases, metabolism decreases, blood viscosity (resistance to flow) increases, and heart rate and cardiac output decrease.[5,20] Uncontrollable shivering and changes in cognitive function may occur, such as confusion, psychosis (loss of reasoning), lethargy, or coma.[5,16,18] Physical signs include facial erythema and edema, ataxia (incoordination of gait), bradycardia, and hypotension.[16]

Treatment of hypothermia takes precedence over frostbite.[20] Passive rewarming or placing the victim in a warm environment (indoors with blankets) is preferred over applying heating pads or immersion in warm baths. Rapid reheating can cause a paradoxical reaction known as "afterdrop," wherein peripheral vasodilatation and subsequent rush of cold fluids from the extremities actually causes core temperature to decrease even further.[16,20] For severe cases of hypothermia, emergency department techniques are required to prevent cardiac fibrillation.[16] Prevention of hypothermia primarily involves avoidance of cold, wet environments and wearing appropriate clothing. Clothes should be layered with a light, wicking material near the skin, insulating materials in the layers in between, and a water-resistant layer on the outside.[5]

Altitude Sickness

Exercise in high altitudes can cause several pathological conditions. Within 6 to 24 hours of ascent to over 12,000 feet, headache, loss of appetite, nausea, irritability, and mild confusion characterizes acute altitude sickness.[21] Although bothersome, this condition is seldom serious at altitudes below 15,000 feet. Most cases resolve in a few days with rest and hydration. Slow ascent to altitude may prevent or substantially decrease symptoms.[18]

Some people experience pulmonary or cerebral edema in high altitude, particularly with rapid ascent to at least 8000 feet.[18,21] Pulmonary edema is recognized by dyspnea, cough, cyanosis, tachycardia, hyperpnea, and rales upon auscultation. Cerebral edema impairs cognitive and other central nervous system functions, causing confusion, ataxia, and loss of consciousness. Early recognition of this serious condition allows descent in a timely manner. Oxygen supplementation and corticosteroids may be needed in more severe cases.[21]

At very high altitude (over 15,000 feet), retinal hemorrhage and retinopathy may occur. Exercise may exacerbate this situation, which is recognized by blurring vision and aching in the orbits. The condition is usually self-limited with no permanent complications if descent occurs quickly.[21]

Metabolic Disorders

Gout

A defect in the breakdown of purine (an amino acid) causes accumulation of uric acid in the blood, a condition called gout. As uric acid concentration increases, it cannot be efficiently excreted by the kidneys and forms crystals in the joints and other tissues. The typical first manifestation of gout is sudden, severe pain and swelling in one or more joints.[6] Over 90% of patients with gout have symptoms in the great toe. The foot, knee, and wrist are also commonly involved. Surgery, fatigue, rich diet, stress, infection, or certain medications can precipitate gout attacks. Chalky, crystal deposits may erupt through the skin of a gouty joint. Unless treated, the attacks recur with increasing frequency and severity, although remissions lasting years are not uncommon.[6] Treatment is through medication and dietary lifestyle changes.

Metabolic Bone Diseases

Osteoporosis

A pathological decrease in bone density (mass per volume) is called osteoporosis.[22] Many factors contribute to the development of osteoporosis, including hormonal disturbances (decreased estrogen), nutritional deficiencies (primarily of calcium), and age.[22] The bones become very fragile and fracture easily. Frequently, compression fractures of the vertebrae cause permanent deformities such as severe thoracic spine kyphosis ("Dowager's hump"), loss of height, and back pain.[22] Simple falls can lead to femur, tibia, humerus, or radius fractures. For persons at risk for osteoporosis (female, postmenopausal, over age 75 years), precautions should be taken when applying manual mobilization techniques, exercising the spine, or performing load-bearing exercises.

Paget's Disease

Paget's disease is an abnormality of bone remodeling, with alternating excess deposition or reabsorption of bone during various stages of the disease.[6] The condition occurs most frequently in the flat and long bones of elderly men.[22] Over time, Paget's disease produces bony deformities, functional disability, head or face pain, and pathological fractures.[6,22] Treatment precautions, such as avoiding heavy loads or extreme motions, are necessary to avoid fracture.

PEDIATRIC CONCERNS

Osteogenesis Imperfecta

Osteogenesis imperfecta (OI) is a congenital condition that affects bone formation.[23] In OI, very brittle bones fracture easily, even during normal weightbearing activity. Persons with OI are nearly always diagnosed in early childhood and rarely participate in athletics. Several variants of OI, from mild to severe, exist and there is no cure.[23] Fractures may be surgically fixated or cast. Most patients become progressively disabled by their multiple fractures and their lifespan is shortened.

SUMMARY

The endocrine system regulates many body functions, normal metabolism, and homeostasis. Pathology of the endocrine glands produces signs and symptoms in many organs, including those of the gastrointestinal, cardiovascular, neurological, urogenital, and musculoskeletal systems. The personal medical history, which can reveal distinct patterns of endocrine dysfunction, is the most important aspect of assessment for endocrine or metabolic disorders. Diabetes, thyroid hormone imbalance (hypo- and hyper-), and Cushing's syndrome (either primary or a result of long-term corticosteroid use) are the most common endocrine disorders. Treatment of endocrine disorders is complicated and may involve many side effects that impair physical activity. Pathological metabolic conditions frequently encountered include adverse environmental exposure (heat, cold, and altitude) and bone diseases. Pathology caused by environmental conditions are treated by prevention (avoiding extreme environments) or removal from the dangerous environment.

RESOURCES

Endocrine-Metabolic

- American Diabetes Association. www.diabetes.org
- atlife.com diabetes and endocrine sites:

  atdiabetes.com/diabetes

  www.atendocrine.com/endocrine
- Yahoo directories:

  dir.yahoo.com/Health/Diseases_and_Conditions/Diabetes/

  dir.yahoo.com/Health/Diseases_and_Conditions/Metabolic_Diseases/

REFERENCES

1. Ganong WF. *Review of Medical Physiology.* 15th ed. Norwalk, Conn: Appleton & Lange; 1991.
2. Gould BE. *Endocrine Disorders. Pathophysiology for the Health-Related Professions.* Philadelphia, Pa: WB Saunders Company; 1997:377-395.
3. Hough DO. Diabetes mellitus in sports. *Med Clin North Am.* 1994;78(2):423-437.
4. Landry GL, Allen DB. Diabetes mellitus and exercise. *Clin Sports Med.* 1992;11(2):403-418.
5. Thein LA. Environmental conditions affecting the athlete. *J Orthop Sports Phys Ther.* 1995;21(3):158-171.
6. Goodman CC, Snyder TEK. Overview of endocrine and metabolic signs and symptoms. In: Goodman CC, Snyder TEK, eds. *Differential Diagnosis in Physical Therapy: Musculoskeletal and Systemic Conditions.* 3rd ed. Philadelphia, Pa: WB Saunders Company; 2000:287-333.
7. Allen DB. Effects of fitness training on endocrine systems in children and adolescents. *Adv Pediatr.* 1999;46:41-66.
8. Boissonnault JS, Madlon-Kay D. Screening for endocrine system disease. In: Boissonnault WG, ed. *Examination in Physical Therapy Practice: Screening for Medical Disease.* New York: Churchill Livingstone; 1995:155-173.
9. Jimenez CC. Diabetes and exercise: the role of the athletic trainer. *Journal of Athletic Training.* 1997;32(4):339-343.

10. Bell DS. Exercise for patients with diabetes: benefits, risks, precautions. *Postgrad Med.* 1992;92(1):183-184,187-190,195-198.

11. Fahey PJ, Stallkamp ET, Kwatra S. The athlete with type I diabetes: managing insulin, diet and exercise. *Am Fam Physician.* 1996;53(5):1611-1617.

12. Martin DE. Glucose emergencies: recognition and treatment. *Journal of Athletic Training.* 1994;29(2):141-143.

13. Petrella RJ. Exercise for older patients with chronic disease. *The Physician and Sports Medicine.* 1999;27(11):79-104.

14. McAllister RM, Delp MD, Laughlin MH. Thyroid status and exercise tolerance: cardiovascular and metabolic considerations. *Sports Med.* 1995;20(3):189-198.

15. Goodman CC. The endocrine and metabolic systems. In: Goodman CC, Boissonnault WG, eds. *Pathology: Implications for the Physical Therapist.* Philadelphia, Pa: WB Saunders Company; 1998:216-262.

16. Bracker MD. Environmental and thermal injury. *Clin Sports Med.* 1992;11(2):419-436.

17. Murray R. Dehydration, hyperthermia, and athletes: science and practice. *Journal of Athletic Training.* 1996;31(2):248-252.

18. Arnheim DD, Prentice WE. Environmental considerations. In: Arnheim DD, Prentice WE, eds. *Principles of Athletic Training.* 8th ed. St. Louis, Mo: Mosby-Year Book; 1993:254-272.

19. Francis K, Feinstein R, Brasher J. Optimal practice times for the reduction of the risk of heat illness during fall football practice in the southeastern United States. *Athletic Training.* 1991;26(1):76-80.

20. Grace TG. Cold exposure injuries and the winter athlete. *Clin Orthop.* 1987;216:55-62.

21. Mountain RD. High-altitude medical problems. *Clin Orthop.* 1987;216:50-54.

22. Boissonnault WG, Bass C. Pathological origins of trunk and neck pain, part III: diseases of the musculoskeletal system. *J Orthop Sports Phys Ther.* 1990;12(5):216-221.

23. Myers GJ. Congenital anomalies: musculoskeletal abnormalities. In: Beers MH, Berkow R, eds. *The Merck Manual of Diagnosis and Therapy.* 17th ed. Whitehouse Station, NJ: Merck Research Laboratories; 1999:2218-2222.

Chapter Eight

Neurological System

PURPOSES

- Describe the basic structures of the neurological system and their functions.
- Review pathophysiological mechanisms of the neurological system.
- Discuss medical history findings relevant to neurological pathology.
- Identify signs and symptoms of neurological pathology.
- Perform physical examination tasks relevant to the neurological system.
- Discuss, compare, and contrast selected pathological conditions of the neurological system.

Figure 8-1. Components of the central nervous system.

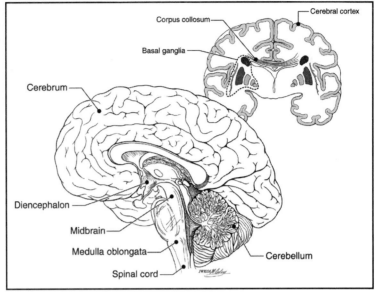

Introduction

The central nervous system (CNS) can be divided (conceptually) into several functional components.[1] The cerebral cortex, basal ganglia, diencephalon (thalamus and hypothalamus), cerebellum, and midbrain-brainstem complex (including the medulla oblongata) compose the brain (Figure 8-1). Table 8-1 lists the relative functions of each section of the brain with respect to motor control. The spinal cord continues the central nervous system from the head to the trunk, carrying neural impulses from the brain to the body and from peripheral receptors to the sensory areas of the brain. The peripheral nervous system begins where nerve roots exit the spinal cord at each vertebral level. Individual peripheral nerves branch out to every organ and system of the body. Much like the vascular system, virtually every cell of the body either receives information from, or provides input to, the nervous system.

Review of Anatomy, Physiology, and Pathogenesis

Cells called neurons comprise the central nervous system. Figure 8-2 shows a typical neuron, including a cell body, dendrites to receive electrochemical input, and one or more axons to carry electrochemical impulses to other neurons. This cell structure varies slightly according to the neuron's location within the nervous system.

Other types of cells serve different functions within the central nervous system. Astroglia, for instance, adhere to blood vessels to form the blood-brain barrier (discussed later). In addition, astroglia assist in regulation of the electrochemical environment necessary for proper neuron function. Microglia cells enter the central nervous system from the blood to remove particles and microbes from the system. Oligodendrocytes bind the neuronal structure together and provide the myelin that surrounds and insulates axons. The astroglia, microglia,

Table 8-1

FUNCTIONAL DIVISION OF THE CENTRAL NERVOUS SYSTEM

Structure	Function
Cerebral cortex	Intentional fine movement control, equilibrium reactions, optic righting
Basal ganglia (within cerebral)	Postural control, gross automatic and fine movements
Diencephalon	Sensory relay and connection with the endocrine system
Cerebellum	Regulates control of posture and movement
Pons-medulla oblongata	Neck and labyrinthine righting reactions, postural response and support reactions
Spinal cord	Reflexes including stretch (myotatic), withdrawal, crossed extension, grasp

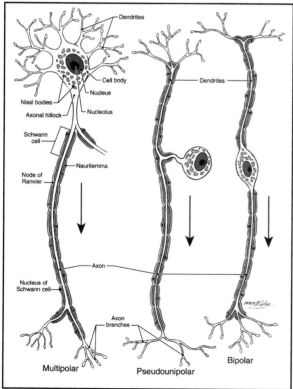

Figure 8-2. General neuron and its structures.

and oligodendrocytes are collectively known as "glial" cells. Ependymal cells form connective tissues that line the cerebral ventricles and central spinal cord canal to contain the cerebrospinal fluid. At various points, the cerebrospinal fluid circulates into the subarachnoid space (see below).

The entire CNS and nerve roots are covered with three connective tissue layers called the meninges. The innermost layer, the pia mater, supports the blood vessels supplying nerve cells and tissues. The arachnoid mater lies immediately above the pia mater. Cerebral spinal fluid circulates between the arachnoid mater and pia mater (the subarachnoid space) to suspend (float) the entire CNS in fluid. The outermost layer is the dura mater, a relatively tough membrane that isolates the CNS from both the internal and external environments.

Blood vessels perfuse the brain, one of the most vascular organs of the body. Under normal circumstances, only certain compounds pass from the blood into the brain. This blood-brain barrier is one of the most important protective mechanisms of the body. Some pathological conditions affect this barrier, subsequently allowing toxic substances into the central nervous system. In addition, the vessels themselves are vulnerable to injury. Damage to these vessels causes hemorrhage within the confined space of the cranium, thus compressing the brain.

The autonomic nervous system, which regulates various body systems and influences behavior, has two components. The sympathetic nervous system increases heart rate, respiratory rate, and neuromotor reaction, usually in response to physical stress such as exercise. The sympathetic system inhibits the gastrointestinal system to avoid diverting blood from working muscles. In contrast, the parasympathetic nervous system functions at rest to regulate basic metabolic processes, such as digestion. It assists recovery from sympathetic stimulation by slowing heart and respiration rates. The opposing but balanced output of these systems plays a major role in homeostasis. The sympathetic responds to internal and external stress, and the parasympathetic restores basal function once the stress is removed.

Signs and Symptoms

Syncope or Coma

Syncope (see Chapter Three), a relatively brief loss of consciousness (lasting seconds or minutes), occurs from a sudden compromise of the brain's vascular supply. *Coma*, however, is a relatively longer state of deep unconsciousness (lasting hours or days), during which the person cannot be aroused to a normal level of consciousness. Coma is rated according to the level of preserved response but never includes conscious control of behavior. Syncope can be the first sign of impending coma, as may occur following head injury and intracranial bleeding.

Paresthesia

Pathology in the nervous system can cause a complete loss of sensation or alter perception of tactile sensation (eg, hyperesthesia, tingling, burning, etc), called paresthesia. The affected body regions are those physically associated with the injured or diseased nerve or neurons.

Abnormal Motor Control, Coordination, or Tone

Decreased deep tendon reflexes, paralysis, weakness, tremors, ataxia, and psychomotor agitation (loss of coordination associated with changes in mood) can be signs of significant neurological system impairment.

Seizure

A sudden electrochemical discharge in the brain, called a *seizure*, can cause a wide range of signs and symptoms.[2,3] Seizures can be partial, affecting only a portion of the brain, or generalized, affecting the majority of the brain.[3] The first of the two major types of seizures is the "petit mal" or "absence" seizure, during which the person briefly loses cognitive awareness and may lose postural control. These seizures often last only seconds and the affected person may not realize a seizure has occurred. During conversation, observers may notice the person pausing in between words or sentences.

The second major type of seizure, the "grand mal" or "tonic-clonic" seizure, causes a sudden, complete loss of consciousness and postural control. The person usually falls to the ground and exhibits extreme postural rigidity (tonic phase) followed by convulsive-type contractions (clonic phase), both involving the entire body.[3] The person may regain consciousness immediately or remain unconscious for some time after seizure activity ceases.[3] Seizures are most often associated with epilepsy, but may also be caused by chemical toxicity, hypoxia, head injury, and other pathological disorders.

Headache

Pain perceived in or around the head is an extremely common symptom associated with many pathological states. Musculoskeletal stress, vascular pathology, or common toxins such as alcohol and nicotine can cause benign headaches (see Chapter Three). An acute headache that persists for several hours is very common following head trauma. Chronic, recurrent, or severe headaches that are not associated with trauma or stress, particularly if increasing in intensity, frequency, or duration, can be a symptom of serious neurological pathology.

Changes in Vision, Hearing, or Other Senses

The senses of smell, sight, hearing, taste, and facial sensation are detected by cranial nerves. Any change in the function of these senses may indicate pathology of the cranial nerves or brainstem (see *Medical History* section for physical examination of the cranial nerves).

Changes in Mental Status

Cognitive changes occur with pathology of the cerebrum, which controls mental function, memory, and personality. Trauma, infection, degenerative or destructive neurological diseases, or biochemical toxicity may induce these changes.

Figure 8-3. Sensory distribution of peripheral nerves.

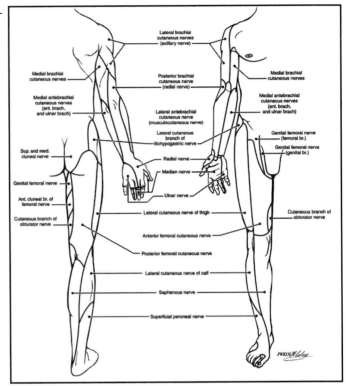

PAIN PATTERNS

Dorsal Spinal Columns

Light touch and proprioception neural impulses travel from the peripheral receptors and nerves to ascend to the brain in the dorsal columns of the spinal cord. These pathways decussate (cross over) in the midbrain to the contralateral cerebrum.

Ventral Spinal Columns

Pain and temperature pathways decussate immediately upon entering the spinal cord and travel up the anterolateral (ventral) columns.

Peripheral Nerves

Specific peripheral nerves transmit sensation, autonomic function, and motor control to specific regions and structures. Figure 8-3 shows sensory distributions of selected peripheral nerves.

Using the above information, the location of lesions within the spinal cord can be approximated. Many neurological diseases affect a specific structure within the nervous system, but some produce lesions in several structures. The distribution of symptoms often aids physicians in preliminary diagnosis, which is confirmed by further clinical, laboratory, and imaging tests.

MEDICAL HISTORY AND
PHYSICAL EXAMINATION

Family and Personal History

Certain neurological conditions, such as epilepsy, muscular dystrophy, and some degenerative central nervous system disorders, have genetic components that may be revealed during a family history. A personal history of neurological pathology may affect physical examination. For example, persons with cerebral palsy would not be expected to have "normal" reflexes or coordination in an affected limb. In addition, medications for such conditions should be noted since they often have many neuromotor side effects.

Inspection

Atrophy of certain muscles suggests peripheral nerve pathology. Certain CNS disorders cause tremors or affect gait and other gross movements. Decorticate and decerebrate posturing indicate lack of communication between the brain (motor cortex and cerebellum, respectively) and the body, a potentially fatal condition. In both, the person falls unconscious and exhibits very rigid, extended legs. The arms may be fixed in flexion (decorticate) or extension (decerebrate).

Physical Examination

Reflexes and Spinal Meningeal Irritation

With practice, the deep tendon reflexes (Achilles', patellar, biceps, and triceps) are easily tested (see Lab Activity 1). The spinal levels of these reflexes, provided in Table 8-2,[4] should be memorized. Asymmetries of reflex amplitude or timing (delay) are important. Athletic trainers document reflexes as "increased" or "decreased" in comparison to the contralateral limb. In rare cases, such as spinal cord injury, a symmetric loss of reflexes distal to the injury can be noted, but the immediate concern is airway management and emergency transportation.

Disruption of the "long motor tracts," which are the cerebral cortex motor neuron pathways, may be assessed with the Babinski test (see Lab Activity 1). Clonus, another abnormal reflex, may be found at the ankle and, occasionally, the wrist. The test is conducted by quickly moving and maintaining the foot (or hand) into end-range dorsiflexion (or extension). A low-amplitude, involuntary oscillation of the foot or hand is abnormal and suggests an upper motor neuron disorder.

Meningeal Irritation

The Kernig and Brudzinski tests for meningeal inflammation are appropriate in cases of suspected meningitis (see Chapter Ten), vertebral disc pathology, or conditions causing inflammation in the spinal canal. Both tests begin with the subject in supine. For the Kernig

Table 8-2

SPINAL LEVELS OF THE DEEP TENDON REFLEXES

Reflex	Spinal Level
Biceps	C5
Brachioradialis	C6
Triceps	C7
Patellar or "knee jerk"	L2 to L4
Achilles' or "ankle jerk"	S1

test, the head is raised either actively or passively. Burning or shooting pain in the spine is a positive sign. The Brudzinski (or "straight leg raise") test involves passively raising one leg at a time, keeping the knee fully extended. At the first sign of pain in the leg or back, the knee is slightly flexed until the symptoms are relieved. The ankle is then passively dorsiflexed, which reproduces the symptoms if meningeal irritation is present. Alternately, the head can be raised after knee flexion, which will again produce symptoms. If dorsiflexion and head flexion do not reproduce the symptoms, the pain is more likely from leg or back muscles. Both tests slightly stretch peripheral nerves and nerve roots, which creates tension on the meninges.

Sensation

Testing sensation on the entire body is usually unnecessary, so the physical examination concentrates around the symptomatic region. Touch sensation travels in bilateral spinal pathways to the brain and is a good, quick test of peripheral nerve and spinal integrity. Sensation, dermatome, and peripheral nerve distributions should be tested separately.

Motor

Similar to the sensory examination, the motor examination is usually limited to the region of injury or symptoms. For nonemergency conditions involving the neck or back, test the upper extremities with suspected cervical problems and the lower extremities with suspected lumbar problems. The motor exam primarily involves testing for myotomal weakness (see Table 1-14).

Balance and Coordination

Balance and coordination tests are usually conducted following head trauma to assess extent of injury or recovery. An athletic trainer may also document the status of a known neuromotor disorder by using such tests.

The Romberg test is used to assess vestibular and postural control. The subject stands relaxed with feet together and eyes closed with the examiner nearby for safety. Loss of balance suggests neurological impairment. Voluntary movement coordination is assessed with two tests. The first involves the person rapidly pointing his or her finger back and forth from his or her nose to a target at arm's length, such as the examiner's finger. This can be done with the eyes open, then repeated with the eyes closed. Inability to contact the target consistently (after some practice) indicates possible cerebellum or basal ganglia disorders. A second coordination test is rapid pronation and supination of both hands, first "in phase" (bilateral simultaneous pronation and supination) and then "out of phase" (one hand pronating while the other supinates). Inability to perform and maintain either task for several seconds indicates a possible cerebellum disorder. If these balance or coordination tests are positive (indicating impairment), further testing by a physician is indicated.

Cranial Nerves

Cranial nerve function indicates the status of the medulla oblongata and can be easily and quickly tested (Table 8-3).[5] Any sign of cranial nerve impairment requires urgent medical referral. If cranial nerve functions are changing rapidly, the situation is a medical emergency.

PATHOLOGY AND PATHOGENESIS

The cerebrum, midbrain, cerebellum, medulla (brain stem), spinal cord, and associated structures (thalamus, hypothalamus, basal ganglia, pons, etc) may be damaged in a number of ways, including trauma, vascular compromise, anoxia, toxicity, and disease (degeneration, cancer, etc). Table 8-4 lists possible etiology and associated signs and symptoms, by structure, for the CNS. While the mechanism can be readily apparent (eg, traumatic blow to the head) or completely unknown, the athletic trainer should recognize signs and symptoms of pathological involvement of the nervous system.

Central Nervous System Disorders

Cerebrovascular Events

Vascular injury (eg, stroke, aneurysm) in the CNS affects the structures supplied by the respective vessels. Signs and symptoms associated with these events appear from the neural region or structures that the vessels supply. In addition, bleeding from these injuries can accumulate in the cranium and compress the brain. Last, blood stimulates an inflammatory response, causing secondary hypoxia in surrounding neural tissue. These events can cause severe, irreversible injury to nerve tissue and may lead to substantial disability. Fortunately they are very rare in younger, active persons.

Brain Trauma

A concussion occurs when the brain collides with the cranium, either at the site of head impact or opposite the site of impact when the brain shifts within the cranium (contrecoup injury).[6] Trauma can temporarily disrupt neural function, alter consciousness or orientation, cause a hematoma in brain tissue, or cause structural damage to neurons. It is important to assess neurological function not only at the time of injury but also at regular intervals for several days. Reevaluation every few minutes for several hours may be necessary in cases of complete loss of consciousness. Reevaluation at least every 15 to 30 minutes for 2 hours and every 4 to 6 hours for 2 days is prudent following a head injury of any severity.

Epidural or Subdural Hematoma

Rupture of cranial or brain blood vessels can cause epidural or subdural hematoma. These conditions develop relatively slowly and may not cause signs or symptoms for up to 24 hours after injury. Parents or roommates should be instructed to check the person's orientation and

Table 8-3

CRANIAL NERVE TESTS

CN	Name	Stimulus	Tests
I	Olfactory	Smell menthol, iso-propyl alcohol	Place odor under the nose (eyes closed). "Tell me what you smell."
II	Optic	Vision acuity and peripheral field	Snellen, Rosenberg charts Cover one eye, wiggle fingers in periphery until they are seen
III IV VI	Oculomotor Trochlear Abducens	Eye movement (all) Pupil control (III)	Follow the finger visually without moving the head to the end of eye motion Pupil reaction with penlight
V	Trigeminal	Face sensation	Sharp, dull sensation on the cheeks
VII	Facial	Face movement	Smile, observe for gross asymmetry
VIII	Vestibulocochlear	Hearing	Rub fingers or crumple paper near the ear
IX X	Glossopharyngeal Vagus	Swallowing	Swallow, watch for tracheal deviation or reported difficulty
XI	Spinal accessory	Shoulder elevation	Resist shrug
XII	Hypoglossal	Tongue movement	Stick out tongue; deviation to one side is abnormal

CN = cranial nerve.

level of consciousness throughout the night. The athletic trainer or a physician should reassess the athlete the following morning. Grading of head injury and return-to-play criteria are well-reviewed elsewhere.[6] Any athlete who has lost consciousness should be withheld from all further participation until neurological testing by a physician has been performed.

Postconcussion Syndrome

Postconcussion syndrome is a spectrum of signs and symptoms that appear or persist for several days or weeks following brain injury. Symptoms include headache, dizziness, attention deficits, and changes in mood. Neurological testing should be conducted to document residual deficits in reflexes, balance, coordination, and mental function. Communicating this information to the treating physician is appropriate. Vigorous physical activity should be avoided until the symptoms resolve completely.

Table 8-4

CENTRAL NERVOUS SYSTEM STRUCTURE, POTENTIAL PATHOGENESIS, AND SIGNS AND SYMPTOMS

Structure	Potential Pathogenesis	Signs and Symptoms
Cerebrum	Cerebral palsy/anoxia, vascular, cancer, trauma, degenerative	Cognition, disorientation, behavioral changes, difficulty initiating movements
Basal ganglia	Vascular, degenerative, cancer	Resting tremor or movements, rigidity, wild and unintentional movements
Midbrain and medulla	Vascular, trauma, multiple sclerosis	Affected breathing and cranial nerve signs
Cerebellum	Vascular, degenerative, trauma	Ataxia, intention tremor, inability to move to target, inability to rapidly alternate movement
Spinal cord	Trauma, vascular, cancer, lateral sclerosis, multiple sclerosis, infection	Weakness/flaccidity, atrophy, hypertonia or hypotonia, or both

In rare instances, acute brain trauma causes an immediate seizure that lasts several minutes. This situation is managed as any other type of seizure (see below), with emergency medical referral.

Cerebral Palsy and Anoxic Brain Injury

An anoxic, metabolic, or ischemic brain injury acquired during birth is called cerebral palsy (CP).[1,7,8] The resulting neurological deficits are not progressive, not communicable, and cannot be transmitted genetically. The most evident and common consequences involve posture and voluntary movement, although sensory, perceptual, or mental disturbances may also occur. Impairment as a result of CP varies depending on the cerebral regions that were damaged. Motor disorders can involve one limb (monoplegia), the unilateral upper and lower extremities (hemiplegia), only the lower extremities (diplegia), or the entire body (tetraplegia).[1,7,8] The most common CP type is spastic, demonstrating hypertonicity (constant spasm). Other types, comprising less than 25% of all cases, include flaccid (hypotonia), ataxic, and dyskinetic (athetoid).[1,7,8]

Athletic trainers may encounter persons with mild or moderate CP in athletics or participating in other physical activities. Adults with CP may have a history of multiple corrective surgeries, overuse injuries, weakness, and impairment of range of motion in affected joints.

Rehabilitation to address CP specifically is usually provided by physical, occupational, and speech therapists.

Epilepsy, Seizure, and Convulsion Disorders

Head injury, drug toxicity, infection, and organic brain anomalies can cause seizure. Many people experience a seizure at some time during their life but do not develop a seizure disorder. A disorder of recurrent seizures is called epilepsy, which has a prevalence of 3% across the population.[2,9] Most people with epilepsy experience seizures before 30 years of age.[2] If an athlete reports a history of epilepsy, the athletic trainer should note the medications and side effects. Most epilepsy medications are tranquilizers and sedatives, which cause drowsiness or incoordination.[9] Epilepsy very rarely causes death, although frequent seizures increase the risk of accidents.

Although many persons with epilepsy do not participate in competitive sports, there is no medical reason why they could not do so.[9] People with epilepsy do not generally appear to be at higher risk for injury during sports than their peers. Exercise may actually inhibit seizures, since most seizures occur at rest rather than during activity.[2] Swimming requires close supervision to avoid accidental drowning. Motor sports are contraindicated for persons who experience one or more seizures per year.[2] Collision and contact sports, however, pose no particular increased risk.[2]

Participation in sports or regular group physical activity may provide psychological benefits. Persons with epilepsy often feel excluded because of their condition and are at increased risk for emotional disturbances and suicide. Being accepted as part of a team or peer exercise group may help allay feelings of exclusion.[2] The athletic trainer should educate coaches and peers as necessary, including the nature of seizures, how to respond to a seizure, and reasonable precautions during activity.

Management of a Seizure

Management of a seizure is first concerned with protecting the person from harm. Removing furniture and bystanders from the immediate vicinity to avoid head or limb injury may be necessary.[9] Towels or pillows can protect the person's head. Nothing should be inserted into the mouth, nor should the mouth be forced open. The person may bite their tongue, become incontinent, or produce copious saliva ("foam at the mouth"). Turning the person on his or her side may prevent blockage of the airway. Once the clonic stage of the seizure ceases, assess airway, respiration, and other vital signs. If clear, begin a secondary evaluation of face, tongue, head, and joints to identify injuries. Upon recovery of consciousness, the person will be confused and should be moved to a quiet area to rest and be reassured.

A first seizure or a seizure lasting more than 5 minutes requires a physician referral. If a seizure does not fit into the person's pattern of previous seizures, a medical referral is appropriate. Any injury incurred during a seizure should be appropriately stabilized and referred to a physician as usual. Discontinuing epilepsy medication often precedes seizures in adolescents.

Spinal Cord Disorders

Spinal Cord Trauma

Traumatic spinal cord injury can be complete, which disrupts all ascending and descending tracts; or incomplete, disrupting only some of the spinal tracts. With complete lesions, all voluntary and autonomic neural functions controlled by neurons distal to the injury are immediately and permanently lost. Function is partially preserved with incomplete lesions depending on the exact site and extent of damage. In addition to the initial structural damage, secondary tissue damage from contusion, inflammation, and compression within the spinal cord follows the acute injury. Some of this secondary damage may be decreased by rapid administration of steroids following the injury. After the acute injury and cessation of neural function distal to the injury (spinal shock), deep tendon reflexes return and spasticity develops. Clonus develops and most autonomic reflexes (eg, bowel and bladder function) return, although sensation and voluntary movement do not.

Spina Bifida

Spina bifida describes congenitally incomplete formation of the neural tube (vertebral arch and meninges) and occurs in various degrees. Meningocele indicates the herniation of the meninges through the defect. Myelomeningocele includes herniation of the spinal cord as well as meninges. Both of these conditions are usually diagnosed at birth and require surgical intervention. Impairment distal to the defect and disability in various degrees result. Other medical complications, such as ventricular swelling and severe scoliosis, occur with these conditions.

Spina bifida occulta, more likely to be encountered by athletic trainers, is the incomplete formation of the posterior vertebral arch without herniation of meninges or the spinal cord.[10] This condition is often discovered upon x-ray for complaints of back pain. Occasionally, skin abnormalities (eg, discoloration, hair, etc) are present over the site of the defect. One or more spinous processes are absent upon palpation. Neurological function (sensation, reflex, or motor) is usually preserved. Treatment for symptomatic cases may require trunk strengthening or, in rare cases, surgical stabilization.

Multiple Sclerosis

Most commonly appearing in early adulthood, multiple sclerosis (MS) forms regions of intermittent inflammation (plaques) in the CNS, causing demyelination of surrounding neurons.[10,11] MS usually affects several regions within the CNS simultaneously (cerebral cortex, cerebellum, and motor and sensory tracts) and follows no standard pattern. The plaques lapse and recur, each recurrence affecting new regions of the CNS. Eventually, demyelination causes irreversible neuronal degeneration.[10]

Signs and symptoms vary depending on where plaques occur in the CNS but commonly include visual disturbances, difficulty speaking (dysarthria), peripheral paresthesia, incoordination, weakness, and unusual fatigue.[10,11] Reflexes may increase, and clonus or the Babinski reflex may appear.[11] The etiology of MS is unknown, although immunologic factors may have a role. Diagnosing MS is difficult and no cure currently exists. Treatment is symptomatic, involving medications to combat inflammation, counseling to avoid fatigue, exercise to preserve function, and speech therapy.[10] Heat seems to exacerbate the symptoms of MS and should therefore be avoided (eg, hydrocollator packs, heated aquatic therapy, etc).

Lifespan is not usually affected (except for cases of severely progressive forms of MS), but impairment and disability may become an issue.[11]

Peripheral Nervous System and Combined Central-Peripheral Disorders

Reflex Sympathetic Dystrophy

Reflex sympathetic dystrophy (RSD) usually occurs in a distal extremity when the CNS produces continuous sympathetic stimulation of a limb.[12] The activity of small-fiber pain receptors from a chronic injury may contribute to development of RSD. Joint injury, limb trauma, lengthy immobilization, disorders affecting nerve roots, and peripheral neuropathy increase risk of RSD.[12,13] In an athletic setting, RSD most commonly develops after a severe injury or fracture that is followed by immobilization and nonweightbearing.

RSD causes symptoms across several peripheral nerve distributions.[12] Symptoms include pain disproportional to the injury, skin hypersensitivity (even to clothes or bed sheets), and extreme reluctance to move the joint or bear weight.[12] Clinical signs include swelling, decreased range of motion, increased skin temperature, and atrophic skin, hair, and nail changes of the affected limb.[12,13] As the syndrome progresses over several weeks, atrophy and poor peripheral vascular control (cyanosis, intolerance to cold, pallor, etc) develops.[12] After several months, sympathetic activity decreases and the entire limb (skin, muscle, and bone) becomes atrophic, cool, pale, and so hypersensitive it is no longer functional.[12,13]

Recognition and treatment of RSD may be very difficult.[12] RSD may be prevented by encouraging movement, particularly at uninjured joints, and progressive weightbearing (if not contraindicated) after an injury. Rehabilitation for RSD consists of rhythmic weightbearing, gentle joint distraction, active range of motion, desensitization techniques, and joint mobilization.[12] Transcutaneous nerve stimulation units may be prescribed for pain relief. Analgesic medications and anesthetic sympathetic blockade injections may also be used in resistant cases.[12] Persistent and aggressive treatment increases the probability of a successful outcome.

Motor Unit and Neuromuscular Disorders

The motor unit is comprised of a single motor neuron, its axon and axon branches (peripheral nerve), and associated muscles fibers. Motor units operate on the "all or none" principle: either the motor neuron discharges and all the associated muscle fibers contract or the neuron fails to discharge and no contraction occurs. Motor unit diseases can affect the motor neuron body, the axons, the neuromuscular junction where the axon joins the muscle fiber, or the muscle itself.[14] Table 8-5 outlines the neurological pathology that affects the various parts of the motor unit.

Motor Neuron

Amyotrophic Lateral Sclerosis

The etiology of amyotrophic lateral sclerosis (ALS or Lou Gehrig's disease) is unknown. ALS occurs in adulthood, most commonly in middle age. Gradual, progressive weakness appears, often noticed first in the hands and arms. Spasticity, hyperactive reflexes, and tics

	Table 8-5
	NEUROMUSCULAR DISORDERS

Structure	Potential Pathology
Motor neuron	Amyotrophic lateral sclerosis (ALS, Lou Gehrig's disease)
	Poliomyelitis and postpolio syndrome
Axon	Peripheral neuropathy
	Guillain-Barré syndrome
Neuromuscular junction	Myasthenia gravis
Muscle	Muscular dystrophy (MD)
	Myopathy, polymyositis, dermatomyositis

develop as the disease progresses, followed by dysarthria and difficulty swallowing (dysphagia). Cognition is unaffected. Treatment is supportive to maintain function as long as possible, including mobility, speech, feeding, and breathing. ALS currently has no cure and half of persons with ALS die within 3 years of onset, although up to 10% will live 10 years. Complications of respiratory failure usually cause death.

Poliomyelitis

Poliovirus destroys motor neurons in the anterior spinal cord, producing the disease called polio (poliomyelitis). Development of effective vaccines and immunization programs has virtually eliminated polio in the United States, although it still occurs in developing countries. The athletic trainer may occasionally encounter someone who recovered from childhood polio. Recovery depends on the amount of motor neuron destruction and strengthening of unaffected motor units.

Postpolio syndrome is very common among polio survivors. This syndrome is characterized by the appearance of symptoms two to three decades after initial infection.[15] Arthralgia, myalgia, weakness, atrophy, and unusual muscle fatigue (and, of course, a history of polio) define postpolio syndrome.[15] The syndrome progresses slowly and is treated symptomatically, with assistive devices and activity modification as necessary.

Axon

Peripheral Neuropathy

Peripheral neuropathy is a generic term describing many disorders of the nerve fiber. Motor and sensory losses occur, as well as loss of vasomotor control. Many different conditions can produce peripheral neuropathy, including diabetes mellitus, trauma, toxicity, infection, or demyelinating disease. Treatment and prognosis for recovery depend on the underlying disorder.

Guillain-Barré Syndrome

An autoimmune response to viral infection most likely causes Guillain-Barré syndrome, an acquired demyelinating polyneuropathy (affecting many nerves). Sudden, disabling symmetric weakness of both legs progresses to the arms and is accompanied by loss of deep tendon reflexes. Cognitive function is maintained, although ability to speak may be affected. Guillain-Barré causes rapid loss of respiratory control and thus requires emergency medical care. Weakness peaks about 3 weeks after onset, but full recovery may take months. In some persons, residual weakness may persist for years and neuropathy may reoccur.

Neuromuscular Junction

Myasthenia Gravis

Myasthenia gravis (MG) is an autoimmune disorder of the neuromuscular junction, where the motor neuron connects to muscle fibers. Extreme muscle fatigue, double vision (diplopia), and ptosis (sagging eyelids) develop suddenly and progressively worsen over several hours or days. Dysarthria, dysphagia, and dyspnea may also occur. Deep tendon reflexes are not affected. Medical treatment consists of corticosteroids and drugs that act at the neuromuscular junction. No cure exists, although most functional ability can be restored and maintained with careful medical management.

Muscle

Muscular Dystrophy

Muscular dystrophy (MD) describes a class of genetic disorders that affects muscle fiber structure. In the most common form—Duchenne's muscular dystrophy—muscle fibers progressively degenerate and are replaced by noncontractile connective tissue. Proximal, limb-girdle (shoulder, pelvis) muscles are affected first, producing wide-base gait, difficulty with stairs, frequent falls, and difficulty rising from the floor. The disease appears in early childhood and wheelchair use is necessary by about 10 years of age. Eventually, the respiratory muscles are affected, usually causing death before the age of 20.

Other forms of MD are less disabling and allow a normal lifespan. No cure for MD exists, although gene therapy has shown promise. Corticosteroids may counter the inflammation accompanying muscle fiber destruction. Moderate exercise to maintain function and nutritional counseling to avoid obesity (which increases demand on muscles) are recommended. Intense physical activity damages muscle and should be avoided.

Management of Neuromotor Diseases

Virtually all diseases of the motor unit adversely affect strength, endurance, and flexibility.[16] Incoordination of posture and voluntary movements may also occur and reflex responses may increase or decrease. Many neuromotor diseases cause progressive weakness and paralysis. Weakness produces limited movement and often leads to secondary problems such as obesity, joint stiffness or contracture, and skin lesions, all of which further inhibit motion and compound the effects of the underlying disease.[16] In addition, metabolic demands of movement and activity increase significantly and may cause fatigue. Aerobic capacity or strength may not increase with rehabilitation exercises, but functional tasks become easier or more effective after conditioning.[16]

Qualification for participation in organized sports is made on a case-by-case basis, depending on the nature and stage of the disease, desired activity and level of competition, approval of the attending physician, and the patient's (or parents') goals. Adaptive sports or activities may be appropriate to protect the participant from injury and allow a rewarding experience. Many of these neuromotor conditions prevent participation in competitive athletics but may occur among physically active individuals.

SUMMARY

Neurological disorders can be obvious or subtle but nearly always affect physical performance. Pathology can occur in any region of the nervous system, including the brain, brainstem, spinal cord, and peripheral nerves. Signs and symptoms depend on the location and extent of the disorder but often include paresthesia, weakness, change in reflexes, incoordination, dysarthria, dysphagia, or dyspnea. Head trauma (concussion and postconcussion syndrome), spinal trauma, and seizure disorders (eg, epilepsy) are the neurological disorders most likely to be encountered among athletes. Many persons with neurological disorders participate in regular physical activity. Athletic trainers should therefore be aware of the basic types of neuromotor disorders and their effects.

RESOURCES

Neurological

- atlife.com neurology site. www.atneurology.com/neurology/
- Neuroland clinical neurology information for professionals. www.neuroland.com (follow the "Health Professional's" link by clicking on the brain)
- Yahoo directory.
  dir.yahoo.com/Health/Diseases_and_Conditions/Neurological_Disorders/

REFERENCES

1. Gould BE. Neurologic disorders. In: Gould BE. *Pathophysiology for the Health-Related Professions.* Philadelphia, Pa: WB Saunders Company; 1997:320-376.
2. Cantu RC. Epilepsy and athletics. *Clin Sports Med.* 1998;17(1):61-69.
3. Fuller KS. Epilepsy. In: Goodman CC, Boissonnault WG, eds. *Pathology: Implications for the Physical Therapist.* Philadelphia, Pa: WB Saunders Company; 1998:785-790.
4. Hoppenfeld S. *Physical Examination of the Spine and Extremities.* Norwalk, Conn: Appleton & Lange; 1976.
5. Goldberg S. *The Four-Minute Neurologic Exam.* Miami, Fla: MedMaster, Inc; 1987.
6. Arnheim DD, Prentice WE. The head and face. In: Arnheim DD, Prentice WE, eds. *Principles of Athletic Training.* 8th ed. St. Louis, Mo: Mosby-Year Book; 1993:680-705.

7. Goodman CC, Miedaner J. Genetic and developmental disorders. In: Goodman CC, Boissonnault WG, eds. *Pathology: Implications for the Physical Therapist*. Philadelphia, Pa: WB Saunders Company; 1998:577-616.

8. Perin B. Physical therapy for the child with cerebral palsy. In: Tecklin JS, ed. *Pediatric Physical Therapy*. Philadelphia, Pa: JB Lippincott Company; 1989:68-105.

9. Arnheim DD, Prentice WE. Other health conditions related to sports. In: Arnheim DD, Prentice WE, eds. *Principles of Athletic Training*. 8th ed. St. Louis, Mo: Mosby-Year Book; 1993:796-819.

10. Gould BE. Congenital and genetic disorders. In: Gould BE. *Pathophysiology for the Health-Related Professions*. Philadelphia, Pa: WB Saunders Company; 1997:97-107.

11. Apatoff BR. Demyelinating diseases. In: Beers MH, Berkow R, eds. *The Merck Manual of Diagnosis and Therapy*. 17th ed. Whitehouse Station, NJ: Merck Research Laboratories; 1999:1473-1476.

12. Kasdan ML, Johnson AL. Reflex sympathetic dystrophy. *Occup Med*. 1998;13(3):521-531.

13. Rosenthal AK, Wortmann RL. Diagnosis, pathogenesis, and management of reflex sympathetic dystrophy syndrome. *Compr Ther*. 1991;17(6):46-50.

14. Homnick DN, Marks JH. Exercise and sports in the adolescent with chronic pulmonary disease. *Adolescent Medicine*. 1998;9(3):467-481.

15. Smith MB. The peripheral nervous system. In: Goodman CC, Boissonnault WG, eds. *Pathology: Implications for the Physical Therapist*. Philadelphia, Pa: WB Saunders Company; 1998:811-837.

16. Small E, Bar-Or O. The young athlete with chronic disease. *Clin Sports Med*. 1995;14(3):709-726.

Chapter Nine

Psychological Conditions

PURPOSES

- Describe basic psychological concepts such as behavior, mood, orientation, and perception.
- Review pathophysiological mechanisms of psychological disorders.
- Discuss medical history findings relevant to psychological disorders.
- Identify signs and symptoms of psychological disorders.
- Perform physical examination tasks relevant to psychological disorders.
- Discuss, compare, and contrast selected psychological disorders.

INTRODUCTION

This chapter discusses several general categories of psychological disorders. The most common psychological issues encountered among athletes are disordered eating and substance abuse. Psychological issues can also affect the course of treatment or the outcome for a musculoskeletal injury. Control of behavior, mood, personality, and cognitive function reside exclusively in the brain. Thus, pathology in the brain can affect psychological status. Psychological disorders may also simulate or mask symptoms from pathology of other organ-systems.

SIGNS AND SYMPTOMS

Change in Sleep Pattern

Psychological disturbance can affect sleep patterns, either increasing or decreasing sleep duration and quality.

Changes in Cognitive Status or Function

Cognitive changes may be noted by the person's family or acquaintances. Increased passivity or aggressiveness, memory problems, inattention or indifference to environment, disorientation in familiar surroundings, or difficulties with ordinary daily tasks (eg, misplacing or losing things, forgetting to turn off appliances, etc) suggest a possible psychological disorder.

Weight Loss and Loss of Appetite

Psychological conditions such as depression and eating disorders can cause significant weight loss or loss of appetite.

Emotional Lability and Changes in Affect (Mood)

Emotional lability refers to frequent, dramatic shifts in mood, such as suddenly switching from uncontrollable laughter to crying. Conversely, pathological changes in affect (mood) are relatively stable, lasting days or weeks. Relatives or friends, rather than the person, often report these changes. People with depression, however, often report "feeling depressed" if specifically asked. The athletic trainer may notice these subtle changes if he or she is familiar with the person.

Unexplainable or Bizarre Symptoms

People with psychological disorders may be unable to describe their perceptions in logical terms. This does not mean, however, that symptoms or injuries are nonexistent. Occasionally, extreme psychological stress (eg, abuse, unstable home environment, extreme emotional or social pressures) causes symptoms that do not correspond with physical examination results. If the clinical presentation (see Chapter One) is not interpretable, referral to a physician with a report of history and physical examination findings is indicated.

PAIN PATTERNS

Somatoform and psychosomatic disorders may produce inconsistent symptoms that do not match any known referral pattern or nerve distribution. Symptoms of pathology in other organ-systems may be exaggerated, misinterpreted, or ignored by someone with a coexisting psychological condition.

MEDICAL HISTORY AND PHYSICAL EXAMINATION

Family and Personal History

Certain psychological conditions, such as depression and substance abuse, have genetic components. A positive family history of a diagnosed psychological condition is significant if behavior or mood changes occur.

Known or reported abuse or social disturbances within the immediate family are major warning signals. As an allied health care professional, the athletic trainer must report suspected abuse to authorities in order to protect the abused person. Obtaining evidence of abuse is very difficult since abused persons often deny their danger. Indicators of child abuse are discussed below.

Many psychotropic medications substantially affect athletic performance and should therefore be documented. Psychotropic medications have various physical side effects. Many affect fine motor coordination and cause weight gain, both of which decrease athletic performance.[1] Furthermore, many of these drugs cause dehydration and hyperthermia,[1] so exercise and fluid intake need to be closely monitored during physical activity.

Physical Examination

Physical examination findings may be inconclusive, confusing, inconsistent, or illogical when a psychological disorder exists. A person's behavior may not indicate psychological status. Persons with significant mental impairment behave erratically, such as walking in circles, muttering the same phrase over and over, or appearing confused or disheveled.[2]

Mental Status Examination

Generally, judging mental function is not in the domain of the athletic trainer, but he or she may recognize mental effects that warrant medical investigation. Table 9-1 lists basic screening questions that can be used to examine mental status.[2,3]

PATHOLOGY AND PATHOGENESIS

The most prevalent psychological issues among athletes are substance abuse and disordered eating.[1,4] Other disorders may arise, either as primary (depression, anxiety, behavioral, and affective disorders) or secondary (following brain trauma) conditions. Table 9-2 outlines

Table 9-1

MENTAL STATUS QUESTIONS

Mental Function	Question	Acceptable Answers or Interpretation
Judgment	If you found a wallet in the lobby of an office building, what would you do with it?	"Turn it in to security" or any other logical answer
Orientation	(Person) What is your name?	Very rarely affected, inability to identify self indicates serious mental impairment
	(Place) Where are you now?	Usually not affected except with serious injury or impairment
	(Time) What quarter/half are we in? What day of the week is it?	Affected even with mild injury or impairment
Cognitive	Subtract backwards from 100 by 7 (or from 50 by 3)	Should be correct for several consecutive series
Memory	List three objects (eg, elephant, hubcap, and pencil) for subject to repeat immediately and at the end of the examination	Remembering any less than all three objects indicates a memory deficit

the general categories of psychological pathology and specific disorders within those categories that are discussed in this chapter. Other than medication side effects or significant disability (eg, requiring hospital care), most psychological conditions do not disqualify someone from participation in sports unless so recommended by a psychiatrist.

Substance Abuse

The current epidemic of substance abuse crosses all gender, socioeconomic, ethnic, and geographical boundaries.[1,4,5] Substance abuse is a pattern of chemical substance use that interferes with normal physiological, social, psychological, or emotional function, or the intentional use of a substance for other than its intended purpose. Any substance that can act biochemically has the potential to be abused, including hallucinogenics, stimulants (eg, amphetamine, ephedrine, caffeine, or phenylpropanolamine), depressants, anabolic steroids, analgesics, narcotics, cocaine, marijuana, caffeine, and over-the-counter medications. Table 9-3 lists signs related to potential drug abuse.

Alcohol and tobacco are the most frequently used and abused drugs in America.[4] The health effects of alcohol (including drunk driving accidents) and tobacco abuse (including several pulmonary diseases) are far greater problems than the consequences of abuse of all other substances combined.[5] Of all drugs, alcohol is the most destructive in terms of preva-

Table 9-2

CLASSIFICATION SCHEME FOR PSYCHOLOGICAL DISORDERS

Category	Specific Disorders
Substance abuse	Prescription or illegal drug abuse, alcoholism
Disordered eating	Anorexia nervosa, bulimia nervosa
Mood disturbances	Depression, bipolar disorder, seasonal affective disorder
Anxiety disorders	Phobias, panic disorders, generalized anxiety, obsessive-compulsive disorder, post-traumatic stress and dissociative disorders
Somatoform disorders	Somatization, hypochondria, conversion disorder, malingering, Munchausen syndrome, chronic pain syndrome
Personality disorders	Antisocial behavior, borderline personality
Psychoses	Schizophrenia, delusional disorders, organic brain syndrome
Child abuse	May coexist with spousal abuse or substance abuse

Table 9-3

BEHAVIORAL SIGNS POTENTIALLY RELATED TO SUBSTANCE ABUSE

- Expresses a feeling or need to limit substance use
- Annoyed by criticism of substance use
- Expresses guilty feelings related to substance use
- Uses substances in morning (eg, for a hangover)
- Uses substances in socially inappropriate situations (eg, during class, practice, work, etc)
- Consistently displays irresponsible behaviors (eg, missed classes, practices, or appointments)
- Increasing academic or legal troubles (eg, declining grades, substance-related arrests)
- Sustains injury as a result of substance use

lence of abuse, social and economic consequences, and medical complications. Anyone drinking alcohol during or before classes, work, or athletic workouts needs immediate intervention and counseling. Such behavior is a sign of uncontrolled alcohol abuse that may lead to alcoholism. Alcoholism (the syndrome of alcohol addiction) is usually treated with abstinence and counseling programs, but has a very high rate of reoccurrence.

Abuse of nicotine in all its forms (cigarettes, cigars, chewing tobacco, snuff, etc) is also a major health concern. Although direct health effects of nicotine are relatively moderate (acting as a mild stimulant), health risks are greatly increased by chronic exposure to the carcinogens introduced by the methods of delivery (eg, inhaled smoke, prolonged contact with oral or nasal epithelium, etc). In addition, since use of most tobacco products is socially acceptable and convenient, nicotine is abused much more frequently than other drugs. This greatly increases the number of exposures over time, which in turn increases the risk of developing disease.

Anabolic steroids, which are the chemical equivalents of the hormone testosterone, receive frequent media attention for abuse among athletes, although many steroid abusers are male adolescents who use them to enhance their physical appearance rather than athletic ability. Medically, anabolic steroids are used to maintain body weight among people with chronic, wasting illnesses. Since no legitimate uses exist for healthy individuals, any use is by definition abuse.

Regular steroid abuse provides muscle mass and strength gains, but also causes side effects including infertility, testicular atrophy, gynecomastia (feminization of the male breast), aggressive behavior, increased libido, and enlargement of the clitoris.[1,5,6] Chronic abuse causes premature epiphysis closure, liver disorders, heart disease, increased blood lipids, and atherosclerosis.[1,5,6] Rapid gain of lean body mass is the most obvious physical sign of anabolic steroid abuse.[6] Stria (stripes of discoloration in the skin), hirsutism, severe acne, hypertension, epistaxis (nose bleed), and needle marks (commonly on the thighs or buttocks) may also be observed.[5,6]

Some athletes abuse stimulants (eg, caffeine, ephedrine, amphetamine, nicotine, etc) to increase physiological excitement.[5] The National Collegiate Athletic Association (NCAA) and International Olympic Committee maintain strict guidelines regarding use of these agents, and outline allowable dosage during athletic competition. Stimulants increase energy and elevate mood, but various side effects can occur: hypertension, tachycardia, hyperpnea, arrhythmia, irritability, hyperthermia, convulsions, coma, and even death.[1,5] Many stimulants are widely available as over-the-counter cold and flu medications, various caffeinated beverages, and certain "health" or "energy" supplements. In high enough doses, any of these substances can be toxic. In addition, most also act as diuretics.

Diuretics increase urine volume, emetics induce vomiting, and laxatives increase defecation. Athletes in sports requiring weight classification (eg, wrestling) or persons with eating disorders may abuse these substances to lose weight.[7] Abuse of these substances can produce dehydration, electrolyte imbalances, and malnutrition, potentially causing an emergency during physical activity.[1]

Unfortunately, abuse of prescription drugs is also frequent. Opiates (narcotics), which are chemical opium derivatives such as heroin, codeine, and morphine, depress the CNS. Opiates are often prescribed as potent analgesics. Abusers of opiates, however, wish to achieve feelings of euphoria (pleasant relaxation). Acute opiate overdose (toxicity) is a medical emergency.[5] Chronic use increases tolerance (increased dose to achieve the same effect) and physical addiction. Sudden cessation after chronic use leads to withdrawal syndromes that can also be life threatening.

Other depressants, such as barbiturates, sedatives, and sleeping pills, cause effects similar to opiates. Low doses produce intoxication and overdose causes depressed breathing, falling blood pressure, and shock. Tolerance, addiction, and withdrawal also occur with abuse of these drugs.

Table 9-4

GENERAL SIGNS OF INTOXICATION
AND WITHDRAWAL SYNDROMES

Intoxication	Euphoria, decreased voluntary motor control, decreased reflex motor control (pupil, deep tendon reflex), behavioral changes (stupor to raging), odor (alcohol, smoke, unusual body odor), poor judgment
Overdose (toxicity)	Hypopnea, syncope, stupor, coma, pinpoint pupils, vomiting, shock
Withdrawal	Tremors, headache, nausea, insomnia, irritability, low-grade fever, diaphoresis

Abuse of illegal drugs, such as marijuana, hallucinogens, cocaine, and heroin, may also be encountered. Heroin, an opiate, is discussed above. Marijuana produces mild intoxication and hallucination, as well as euphoria, tachycardia, and hypertension.[5] Other hallucinogens, such as LSD, are also frequently abused. The relative toxicity of these drugs is generally low (ie, require large doses for a toxic effect), but their purity may be questionable. Other substances used to "cut" or dilute the drug to obtain a greater number of doses increases their danger. Hallucinogens affect behavior and cognitive processing, which can increase risk of accidents when performing other activities requiring coordination or judgment.

Cocaine, extracted from the coca leaf, acts as a stimulant in the body. It can be absorbed through oral (chewed leaves) or nasal (snorted powder) membranes, intravenous injection, or through the alveoli by inhalation of smoke vapor.[5] Cocaine ingestion can cause acute hypertension, tachycardia, irritability, seizure, cardiac arrhythmia, and coronary artery spasm (leading to myocardial infarction).[5] Smoking marijuana, cocaine, or heroin can also lead to inflamed, obstructed airways, similar to cigarette smoking.

Risk of cardiac death during exercise is increased after using drugs such as cocaine, anabolic steroids, and alcohol.[8-12] Specifically, cocaine can induce coronary artery spasm, and anabolic steroids can cause hypertrophic cardiomyopathy.[9,12] Drug abuse can also cause myocardial ischemia, inflammation, or fibrosis, as well as a host of other medical complications.[8,11]

Table 9-4 lists the general signs of intoxication, overdose, and withdrawal. Most cases of mild intoxication, depending on the drug, can be treated by removal to a quiet room, reassurance, and rest. If changes of vital signs occur, immediate emergency medical care is needed. Overdose, or toxicity, of any drug is a medical emergency and should be managed as such. Maintaining airway and breathing take precedence, and transportation to a medical facility is indicated. Withdrawal, a physical and psychological condition, occurs following the cessation of a physically addicting substance after chronic abuse. Withdrawal from physically addictive drugs (ie, alcohol, opiates, sedatives, and barbiturates) can be fatal and should be medically supervised. Treatment of substance abuse requires substantial physical and psychological intervention and social support.

Eating Disorders versus Disordered Eating

A distinction exists between a medically diagnosed eating disorder and the syndrome of disordered eating, although the two conditions are associated.[13] Many athletes, particularly female athletes, display behaviors described as disordered eating, including restrictive diets (fad or extreme diets) or occasional binge-eating (excessive intake of food) and purging (self-induced vomiting or excessive laxative use). Frequency of disordered eating increases with female gender (10 to 1 female to male ratio), perfectionist personality, abnormal attention to body image, participation in sports emphasizing a thin body (eg, gymnastics or figure skating), sports associating low body fat with success (eg, running or swimming), or sports that classify participants by weight category (eg, wrestling, boxing, or martial arts).[1,13-16] Long-term dieting (particularly during adolescence), significant emotional trauma (injury, change in coach, family problems, etc), and substantial increases in training load have also been implicated in disordered eating among elite female athletes.[16] Other psychosocial factors are often discovered after development of disordered eating, such as a conflicted family environment, physical or sexual abuse, inability to handle stress, low self-esteem, and personality disorders.[13,16,17]

Disordered eating often begins as seemingly harmless dieting, such as eliminating meat or "fattening foods" to lose weight. Over time, however, a self-imposed "forbidden foods" list is created.[13] Simultaneously, exercise increases to excessive levels, often consuming several hours a day. Obsessive and compulsive behaviors eventually become associated with other daily routines.

The person may criticize other people's eating behaviors or begin to purge (induce vomiting) in addition to restricting his or her diet.[13] Alternately, the person may binge (consume large quantities of food) in reaction to severe hunger, then purge in response to feelings of guilt.[13] Weight loss, dry skin, brittle nails, intolerance to cold, menstrual disorders, orthostatic hypotension, dizziness, and constipation may be early signs of disordered eating. Indications of frequent vomiting, such as fatigue, sore throat, abdominal pain, edematous face, and sour breath may also appear.[13] Dehydration and inadequate caloric intake increase the risk of injury or illness while participating in physical activity.[7]

If these behaviors persist, the probability of developing an eating disorder increases dramatically. The most common eating disorders among active people are anorexia nervosa and bulimia nervosa.[13,14,17] Anorexia nervosa has been noted in 5% to 15% of young females with amenorrhea (and approximately 1% of all females), with reported mortality as high as 10% to 20%.[15,17] The hallmark signs of anorexia nervosa are severely underweight appearance, inability to recognize self-emaciation, and refusal to maintain body weight within an acceptable range for height and gender.[7,17] Avoidance of weight gain becomes an obsession and a substantial distortion of body image develops. Among females, malnourishment eventually produces amenorrhea (see Chapter Seven).[7,15,17]

Anorexia nervosa is often episodic (ie, cycles of remission and recurrence), with severity of behavior increasing in each successive episode.[13] Persons with anorexia nervosa may purge, use laxatives, or use diuretics to avoid weight gain. Despite multiple metabolic crises, persons with anorexia often continue to exercise compulsively to excess.[13,17] Anorexia nervosa, if untreated, causes electrolytic imbalances, dehydration, endocrine dysfunction, cardiovascular disorders, metabolic collapse, and eventually death from starvation or cardiac failure.[7]

Bulimia nervosa is characterized by "binge and purge" cycles recurring at least twice a week for 3 consecutive months.[15] Binge-eating is defined by bouts of rapid and massive food

Table 9-5

WARNING SIGNS FOR EATING DISORDERS

- Obsession with calories and body weight
- Expression of "being fat" when in fact he or she is not
- Consuming inappropriate amounts of food, high or low
- Compulsive exercise
- Expresses concern about other people's eating
- Greater than 5% change in body weight in 4 weeks
- Sudden changes in mood or personality

intake, up to 10,000 or 15,000 calories in less than 2 hours.[13,17] To avoid weight gain, purging occurs shortly after binge-eating. Most commonly, purging manifests as self-induced vomiting. Other purgative behaviors include laxative and diuretic abuse (although neither affects caloric absorption), excessive exercise, or self-imposed fasting.[7,13,15,17] Purging is associated with many complications, including electrolyte imbalances, gastrointestinal disturbance, renal complications, and seizures.[7,18]

In contrast to anorexia nervosa, persons with bulimia nervosa often have normal body weight and do not develop amenorrhea. They express concern about their "lack of control" over eating or food, whereas persons with anorexia exhibit very strict control of their eating habits. An estimated 1% to 3% of young women have bulimia nervosa, which has a lower mortality than anorexia nervosa.

Abrasions or lacerations on the back of the hand or knuckles ("Russell's sign") may be the most obvious physical sign of bulimia nervosa.[18] These lesions are created during self-induced vomiting as the upper incisors cut the dorsum of the hand.[18] Associated physical findings are erosions of the posterior surface of the frontal teeth and inflamed parotid glands (anterior and inferior to the ears), but these lesions are more difficult to observe.[7,18]

Treatment of eating disorders has two components: recognition and intervention.[15] Recognizing eating disorders may be difficult unless the associated behaviors are directly observed. Table 9-5 lists warning signs of disordered eating syndromes.[7,13,15,19,20] Intervening when disordered eating is suspected can also be difficult, requiring a desire to understand rather than accuse.[13] Presenting evidence of the behaviors and expressing concern for health are appropriate first interventions.[13] Involving family members or friends in a nonconfrontational manner may be necessary. If an eating disorder is suspected, referral to a physician and a multidisciplinary treatment program are required.[15,17,21]

Prevention programs, particularly among young female athletes, may be useful. Effects of disordered eating on health and athletic performance should be presented.[14] In addition, education of coaching staff to avoid comments or behaviors that may inadvertently reinforce disordered eating may be appropriate.[15] The NCAA and the National Athletic Trainers' Association (NATA) provide information for such educational programs.

Mood Disorders

The major "mood disorders" (formerly called "affective disorders") include depression, bipolar disorder, and seasonal affective disorder.

Table 9-6

SIGNS OF INCREASED SUICIDE RISK

- Depression
- Substance abuse
- Previous suicide attempt
- Recent personal loss
- Family history of suicide
- Expression of hopelessness
- Social isolation
- Impulsive or secretive behavior

Depression

Prevalence of depression, a medical condition wherein feelings of grief or sadness impair physical and social function, is estimated to be between 10% and 20%.[22] Signs and symptoms include loss of pleasure, changes in body weight (gain or loss), disturbed sleep pattern, fatigue, inability to concentrate, and suicidal thoughts or expressions.[22] Behavioral manifestations include isolation from family and friends, sudden changes in academic or athletic performance, interpersonal conflicts, and increased complaints of medical problems.[22] Depression is a major risk factor for suicide. Table 9-6 lists other suicide risk factors.[23-25]

Bipolar Disorder

Recurrent cycles of depression and abnormal elation (mania), severe enough to impair normal daily life characterizes bipolar disorder.[2] The signs and symptoms of the depression phase are similar to those listed above. The elation, or manic phase, produces hyperactive motor and speech patterns and insomnia. During this phase the person may be very productive. Eventually, however, this overstimulated state interferes with judgment and social interactions.[2]

Seasonal Affective Disorder

Seasonal affective disorder describes depression that occurs only during particular seasons, most commonly during winter months.[26,27] The condition completely resolves during the other seasons. Increased sleep, food intake, weight gain, irritability, and mild physical fatigue occur in seasonal affective disorder.[26,27] More common among females (4 to 1 ratio) in early adulthood and decreasing with age, it often occurs in northern latitudes because of more pronounced seasonal sunlight and weather changes. As with depression, seasonal affective disorder may affect performance.[26] Depression, seasonal or otherwise, requires referral to a physician or psychological health consultant. Artificial light exposure of a certain intensity and duration is often used as treatment, although medication or psychotherapy may be used to augment treatment.[26,27]

Anxiety Disorders

Perceived physical, mental, or emotional stress normally causes anxiety, a state of intense worry. Pathological anxiety, however, changes behavior (eg, avoidance) or interferes with normal social function. Several types of anxiety disorders are identified: phobias, obsessive-compulsive disorders, and dissociative disorders.[2]

Phobias

Abnormal fear of a specific object or situation that does not cause anxiety in the average person is a phobia.[2] A common example among athletes is performance anxiety, where the phobia may become so intense that performance is impaired or avoided. Clinical indications of a phobia (other than emotional anxiety) may include physical avoidance of a situation or object, increased psychoemotional stress upon mention or thought of a situation or object, or unusual attachment to a "protective" person or place.[22]

Generalized anxiety disorder, another example of phobia, is characterized by incessant worry about future events, self-conscious mannerisms, perfectionist attitude, and desire for constant reaffirmation from others.[22] Panic attacks, which are episodes of frequent and intense anxiety, impair daily life.

Obsessive-Compulsive Disorder

Recurrent disabling thoughts that are centered on an irrational or unreasonable fear constitute an obsession. Compulsions are behaviors that are repeated ritualistically, sometimes hundreds of times a day.[28] Persons with obsessive-compulsive disorder display related obsessions and compulsions, such as a compulsion to recheck a locked door because of an obsession with being robbed. When these behaviors interfere with daily life, the condition may require treatment with medication and counseling. Depression commonly coexists in persons with obsessive-compulsive disorder.[28]

Dissociative Disorders

Dissociative disorders occur when a person's identity or behavior suddenly changes so radically that "association" (or memory) of their "former self" is temporarily lost.[23] People with dissociative disorders often have no awareness of their alternate identities. Dissociative disorders can be induced by extreme physical-behavioral stress (a form of post-traumatic stress syndrome), such as prolonged physical or mental abuse, severe injury, or extreme emotional states.[29]

In such situations, the mind separates intolerable thoughts and experiences from the primary identity by forming alternate identities. These identities experience and remember the situation, thus sparing the primary identity. Complete amnesia for a single event or period of time may exist, or entirely separate personalities may develop if the offending experiences are recurrent or unresolved (ie, repetitive physical or sexual abuse, overwhelming debt). Treatment is complex, involving medication and extensive psychotherapy in order to reintegrate the person's identity. Addressing the experiences that led to dissociation is a focus of treatment.[29]

Somatoform Disorders

Somatoform disorders are perceived or imposed physical disorders produced by mental or emotional disturbances. The person unconsciously seeks attention and comfort for an imagined, exaggerated, or artificially imposed physical problem. Complaints are often vague, exaggerated, inconsistent, and recurrent.[22] The family or home environment may be a factor in these syndromes, including overprotective spouse or parents, frequent but unresolved family conflicts, a major life event (divorce, death of a family member), or physical or sexual abuse.[22] An athletic trainer should never assume a somatoform disorder exists. If the person's comments or behavior suggest a psychological issue, medical referral with complete documentation is indicated.

Personality Disorders

Personality disorders may appear as recurrent antisocial behaviors, such as violence or crime.[22] Often, the behavior continues to escalate in frequency and severity despite disciplinary efforts. A type of personality disorder is "borderline" personality, or abnormal dependence on other people for personal psychoemotional stability. Similar to other major psychological illnesses, an unstable or abusive family environment can contribute to development of an unstable personality.

Psychoses

Psychoses are disorders of orientation to physical surroundings. The ability to perceive and interpret experiences and surroundings is impaired. Persons who have psychotic disorders may hallucinate (visual, auditory, or sensory) or display a complete lack of logical order to their thoughts and actions. Psychoses are extremely disabling and therefore rarely encountered in competitive athletics.

PEDIATRIC CONCERNS

Child Abuse

Child abuse is a familial or social disorder, meaning that the entire family is affected by the illness. Any behavior that interferes with a child's development, particularly one that results in changes in the child's personality, is child abuse.[2] In many cases, the abused child acts like an adult and becomes a "caretaker" for other family members.[2] Aggressive behavior appears and increases in frequency, but the abused child may seem unaware (or indifferent) of the effects of violence.[2] The family often isolates itself socially and physically, avoiding contact with relatives and authority figures. The parents often express very high expectations for the child, and may rely on the child for emotional support.[2,30]

Various manifestations of child abuse include physical, sexual, emotional, or neglect (withholding physical and emotional support), with neglect being the most commonly reported. Neglect is associated with parental substance abuse or depression, which affects the parent's ability to care for both him or herself and his or her family.[30]

The family situation can be very complex in the case of an abused child, usually including one abusive parent and one who "looks the other way," is abused themselves, or is completely passive in family interactions. More than one sibling may be abused, and often the abusive parent was abused as a child and consequently failed to develop emotionally.[30] In addition, an abused child may be hyperactive, impulsive, or handicapped, thus requiring more emotional support than the parents are capable of providing. The abusive parent resents the dependency of the disabled child, which reinforces the abusive behavior.

Identifying child abuse is complicated. Suspicion should be raised under certain circumstances. A parent or child unable or unwilling to report a mechanism of injury, or an injury that is inconsistent with the history, may be early indications.[30] Signs of abuse include skin injuries (cuts, bruises, burns) hidden under clothing, abdominal trauma, face and head trauma, or a fracture without a reasonable history. Most suggestive of abuse are multiple injuries in various stages of healing.[30]

Signs of neglect include malnutrition, fatigue, poor hygiene, poor school attendance, and trouble with peer social interactions.[30] Discussions with the child and parents should be calm and supportive, attempting to elicit information rather than making accusations.[30] Treatment may involve medical treatment of injuries, removing the child from the family, family counseling, and long-term family therapy.[30]

Health care workers are required by law to report suspected abuse to local child and family protection agencies but may feel reluctant to do so without "hard evidence." Careful documentation is essential, including history, physical examination findings, and notes of parental meetings or discussions if possible. State and local laws regarding the reporting of child abuse should be familiar. The regulations often include what required information and specific situations obligate reporting to a protective agency.

Behavioral or Conduct Disorders

Behavioral or conduct disorders among children and adolescents may be indicative of psychological or social disturbances.[2,22] Recurrent, escalating violent or antisocial behavior (fighting, vandalism, setting fires, stealing, etc.) may be a result of an unstable or abusive home environment, poor adult role models, lack of parental empathy or contact, or substance abuse by the family or child.[2,22] A limited sense of responsibility or consequences of behavior and a decreased ability to learn from experience develops.[22] When confronted, the child may blame his or her behavior on others (eg, "they left me no choice").[22] Treatment with medication decreases aggressive behavior. Various psychosocial interventions, including family psychotherapy, peer group programs, and psychological counseling, address other contributing psychosocial issues.[22]

SUMMARY

Psychological disorders, while relatively common, may be very difficult to detect and may or may not affect physical performance. Mental, social, or emotional impairment is often as disabling as physical impairment. Understanding psychological disorders may assist the athletic trainers when they work with people who have these conditions. Changes in mood or behavior may accompany onset of a psychological disorder. Unstable family or home life also contributes to development of many psychological conditions. Disordered eating, substance abuse, and child abuse are psychological conditions that may be encountered in sports medicine settings.

RESOURCES

Psychological

- atlife.com psychology/psychiatry site. www.atpsychiatry.com/psych/

- Yahoo directories:

    dir.yahoo.com/Health/Diseases_and_Conditions/Eating_Disorders/

    dir.yahoo.com/Health/Diseases_and_Conditions/Mental_Health/

REFERENCES

1. Macleod AD. Sport psychiatry. *Aust N Z J Psychiatry.* 1998;32:860-866.

2. Good WV, Nelson JE. *Psychiatry Made Ridiculously Simple.* 2nd ed. Miami, Fla: MedMaster, Inc; 1991.

3. Goldberg S. *The Four-Minute Neurologic Exam.* Miami, Fla: MedMaster, Inc; 1987.

4. Blood KJ. Non-medical substance use among athletes at a small liberal arts college. *Athletic Training.* 1990;25(4):335-338.

5. Felter RA, Fitzgibbon J. Drug-related emergencies in athletes. *Clin Sports Med.* 1989;8(1):129-138.

6. Potteiger JA, Stilger VG. Anabolic steroid use in the adolescent athlete. *Journal of Athletic Training.* 1994;29(1):60-64.

7. Stephenson JN. Medical consequences and complications of anorexia nervosa and bulimia nervosa in female athletes. *Athletic Training.* 1991;26(2):130-135.

8. Basilico FC. Cardiovascular disease in athletes. *Am J Sports Med.* 1999;27(1):108-121.

9. Franklin BA, Fletcher GF, Gordon NF, et al. Cardiovascular evaluation of the athlete: issues regarding performance, screening and sudden cardiac death. *Sports Med.* 1997;24(2):97-119.

10. Futterman LG, Myerburg R. Sudden death in athletes: an update. *Sports Med.* 1998;26(5):335-350.

11. Maron BJ. Cardiovascular risks to young persons on the athletic field. *Ann Intern Med.* 1998;129(5):379-386.

12. O'Connor FG, Kugler JP, Oriscello RG. Sudden death in young athletes: screening for the needle in a haystack. *Am Fam Physician.* 1998;57(11):2763-2770.

13. Johnson MD. Disordered eating in active and athletic women. *Clin Sports Med.* 1994;13(2):355-369.

14. Dick RW. Eating disorders in NCAA programs. *Athletic Training.* 1991;26(2):136-147.

15. Grandjean AC. Eating disorders: the role of the athletic trainer. *Athletic Training.* 1991;26(2):105-112.

16. Sundgot-Borgen J. Risk and trigger factors for the development of eating disorders in female elite athletes. *Med Sci Sports Exerc.* 1994;26(4):414-419.

17. Johnson C, Tobin DL. The diagnosis and treatment of anorexia nervosa and bulimia among athletes. *Athletic Training.* 1991;26(2):119-128.

18. Daluiski A, Rahbar B, Meals RA. Russell's sign: subtle hand changes in patients with bulimia nervosa. *Clin Orthop.* 1997;343:107-109.

19. Teitz CC, Hu SS, Arendt EA. The female athlete: evaluation and treatment of sports-related problems. *J Am Acad Orthop Surg.* 1997;5(2):87-96.

20. West RV. The female athlete: the triad of disordered eating, amenorrhea, and osteoporosis. *Sports Med.* 1998;26(2):63-71.

21. Woscyna G. Nutritional aspects of eating disorders: nutrition education and counseling as a component of treatment. *Journal of Athletic Training.* 1991;26(2):141-147.

22. Post D, Carr C, Weigand J. Teenagers: mental health and psychological issues. *Prim Care.* 1998;25(1):181-192.

23. Bilkey WJ, Koopmeiners MB. Screening for psychological disorders. In: Boissonnault WG, ed. *Examination in Physical Therapy Practice: Screening for Medical Disease.* 2nd ed. New York: Churchill Livingstone; 1995:277-301.

24. Schapira K. Suicidal behavior. In: Beers MH, Berkow R, eds. *The Merck Manual of Diagnosis and Therapy.* 17th ed. Whitehouse Station, NJ: Merck Research Laboratories; 1999:1544-1549.

25. Smith AM, Milliner EK. Injured athletes and the risk of suicide. *Journal of Athletic Training.* 1994;29(4):337-341.

26. Rosen LW, Smokler C, Carrier D, et al. Seasonal mood disturbances in collegiate hockey players. *J Athl Training.* 226;31(3):225-228.

27. Saeed SA, Bruce TJ. Seasonal affective disorders. *Am Fam Physician.* 1998;57(6):1340-1346.

28. Goodman CC. Biopsychosocial concepts related to health care. In: Goodman CC, Boissonnault WG, eds. *Pathology: Implications for the Physical Therapist.* Philadelphia, Pa: WB Saunders Company; 1998:9-43.

29. Kluft RP. Dissociative disorders. In: Beers MH, Berkow R, eds. *The Merck Manual of Diagnosis and Therapy.* 17th ed. Whitehouse Station, NJ: Merck Research Laboratories; 1999: 1519-1525.

30. Sayre JW. Child abuse and neglect. In: Beers MH, Berkow R, eds. *The Merck Manual of Diagnosis and Therapy.* 17th ed. Whitehouse Station, N.J.: Merck Research Laboratories; 1999: 2300-2303.

Immunology

PURPOSES

- Describe the basic physiology of immunology.
- Review pathophysiological mechanisms of immunology, including contributions to homeostasis.
- Describe the effect of exercise on immunology.
- Discuss medical history findings relevant to immune system pathology.
- Identify signs and symptoms of immune system pathology.
- Perform physical examination tasks relevant to the immune system.
- Discuss, compare, and contrast selected immune pathology.

Table 10-1

TYPES OF INFECTIOUS ORGANISMS

Type	Structure	Mode of Replication	Environmental Factors
Bacteria	Simple single-celled organisms	Replicate independent of host	Do not depend on host for survival
Viruses	Non-cellular genetic strands	Use host's internal cellular mechanisms to replicate	Cannot exist outside the biological environment of the host(s)
Parasites (protozoa)	Complex single-celled organisms with multiple or undifferentiated cells	Replicate independent of host	Exist in the environment and the host
Fungi (mycoses)	Primitive single-celled plants, commonly yeasts and molds	Replicate by spores	Dependent on host and environment for growth (but not necessarily for reproduction)

INTRODUCTION

Infection is the immune system's response to invasion of the body by viruses, bacteria, fungi, or parasites (Table 10-1). The immune system involves the skin, mucous membranes, bone, blood, and lymph. Physical, behavioral, psychological, environmental, and nutritional factors can all affect immune system function.[1] Contact with infected tissues or body fluids, contact with contaminated objects or substances, or inhaling airborne microbes are methods of person-to-person exposure to infectious organisms.[2] Athletes may be at increased risk for infection because of frequent travel, close physical contact with other individuals, sharing of facilities and equipment, and altered sleep patterns, all of which suppress the immune system's responses.[1]

A host is a person (or animal) that harbors an infectious organism. In general, infectious organisms perpetuate themselves by passing from host to host. Life cycles of some infectious organisms include a vector, often an insect, that transmits the disease-causing organism between hosts. The vector is usually not affected but may pass the infectious organism to many hosts. Infectious diseases that can pass person-to-person without vectors are called contagious. Communicable diseases, however, can be passed from any animal to any other, and thus include vector-mediated diseases. This chapter reviews some common infections of various organ systems that may be encountered among physically active people.

REVIEW OF PHYSIOLOGY AND PATHOGENESIS

Table 10-2 outlines the two components of the immune response: the general response and responses specific to the invading microbe.[3] Within these responses are the humoral

Table 10-2 COMPONENTS OF THE IMMUNE RESPONSE		
Component	General	Specific
Humoral (bloodborne)	Protein complement	Immunoglobins (antibodies)
Cell	Phagocytosis (macrophages, monocytes)	B-cells, T-cells

(activated protein "complement" and immunoglobins circulating in the bloodstream) and cell-mediated (activated immune system cells) mechanisms.[4]

The immune system includes the physical barriers of the skin and mucous membranes, the acidic environment of the body, and phagocytic cells in the bloodstream.[4,5] The general response alters metabolism to mobilize energy sources and nutrients to meet the increased demands of infection.[3] Substances released from macrophages, monocytes, and T-cells (cell-mediated general response) activate protein complement in the blood, which binds foreign particles (humoral general response).[4,5] This occurs during the fever phase in proportion to the virulence (aggressiveness) of the infection.[3,4]

The cell-mediated specific response involves activated T-lymphocytes (T-cells) and B-lymphocytes (B-cells). This response is stimulated by antigens, which are proteins on the outer cell wall of invading microbes.[4] The B-cells then produce immunoglobins, which are complex immune proteins that form antibodies specific to the invading antigen, thus providing the humoral specific response. These antibodies allow phagocytes to recognize and destroy a foreign microbe. The B-cells "remember" antigens and secrete the appropriate antibodies when subsequently stimulated by antigens of the same infectious organism.[4,5] Thus, T-cells are critical to immune function since they regulate B-cell activity and stimulate the general immune responses.[4] Table 10-3 lists immune responses to the various types of invading organisms.

The generalized response causes muscle catabolism, which releases proteins to convert into energy (through gluconeogenesis) and supplies amino acids for white blood cells to combat infection.[3] Fast-twitch muscle fibers, followed by slow-twitch and finally cardiac muscle, are affected. Inhibition of muscle energy (oxidative and glycolytic) pathways impedes aerobic and strength performance. Insulin level increases to enhance glucose uptake and fat metabolism is inhibited.[3]

During recovery from infection, strength remains limited until muscle protein is replaced, usually in 2 to 4 weeks. Aerobic function, however, is significantly affected by decreases in blood volume (dehydration), hemoglobin, cardiac efficiency, and muscle mass, and may not recover for up to 3 months.[3]

Effect of Exercise on Immune Function

Prolonged, intense exercise (such as marathon training) suppresses the immune system.[6] These temporary changes, however, may not increase the risk of infection.[1,7] Moderate exercise actually appears to have a slight beneficial effect on the immune system.[7,8] Physical and

Table 10-3

RESPONSE OF THE IMMUNE SYSTEM
TO VARIOUS INVADING ORGANISMS

Microbe	*Immune Response*
Bacteria or fungi	Macrophages; T-cells stimulating neutrophils (general, cell-mediated), some B-cell and antibody action
Parasites	Macrophages stimulate T-cells to stimulate eosinophils (general, cell-mediated); B-cells, particularly if toxins are produced by a parasite; some humoral mechanisms
Viruses	Macrophages stimulate T-cells to stimulate "killer" cells and cytotoxic T-cells; B-cells and some humoral proteins are effective for some viruses

emotional stresses are catabolic, damaging musculature and other organs that release metabolic byproducts (eg, acids, "free radicals"). The immune system response to these metabolic byproducts potentially depletes resources available to fight infection if exercise is excessive.[6,7]

Exercise in the presence of an active infection may be contraindicated.[3] Most bacterial infections do not worsen, but viral and parasitic infections nearly always increase in severity with exercise.[4] In addition, viruses may migrate to additional organs and tissues, such as the myocardium. Regardless of the invading organism, athletic performance nearly always decreases.[4] Chest pain, tightness, or palpitations requires rest from athletics until fever and other symptoms resolve.[3] Since determining whether an infection is bacterial or viral is impossible without medical tests, the athletic trainer should recommend rest from physical activity if fever is present.

SIGNS AND SYMPTOMS

Most infections cause fever and produce pain and edema in the affected organ or system, resulting in signs and symptoms specific to that system. Hence, the signs and symptoms relevant to each system should be reviewed (Chapters Three through Eight).

Fever

Fever can generally be classified as "low-grade" (less than 102°F) and "high grade" (102°F and above). While both indicate pathology, high-grade fever suggests a more serious illness. Sustained body temperature over 104°F kills brain cells and may cause irreversible cell necrosis in other organs. Fever can also induce arthralgia, myalgia, anorexia, fatigue, and diaphoresis.

Fatigue

Metabolic rate increases with infection. Increased energy demand and catabolism of muscle and other tissues cause a progressive and persistent fatigue.

Lymphadenitis

Swelling of the lymph nodes (lymphadenitis) indicates infection. The infection is usually distal to the swollen lymph nodes.

Localized Pain, Redness, Heat, and Swelling

Signs of inflammation occur with infection and are easily observed when superficial tissues are affected.

Unusual Muscle and Joint Pain

Infection may cause muscle or joint pain that does not change with movement and becomes progressively worse over time.

PAIN PATTERNS

An infection produces signs and symptoms related to the system it affects. Secondary signs and symptoms may arise as additional associated systems become infected.

MEDICAL HISTORY AND PHYSICAL EXAMINATION

Family and Personal History

Personal history may reveal symptoms consistent with infection, such as fever, fatigue, arthralgia, or myalgia. The course of the symptoms is important, including origin, intensity, and duration.

Inspection and Physical Examination

Purulent (containing pus) drainage from a wound, eye, ear, nose, mouth, nipples, urethra, or anus virtually ensures an infection exists within those structures. Likewise, erythema and edema in joints and deep body tissues indicate inflammation, possibly caused by an infection. Lymphadenitis or other palpable masses within body tissues, particularly if tender, suggest infection.

PATHOLOGY AND PATHOGENESIS

Upper Respiratory Infections

Several types of virus produce upper respiratory infection (URI).[4,8-10] For example, most common colds (coryza) are the result of rhinovirus infection.[8,10] URI produces various signs and symptoms, including rhinitis, rhinorrhea, sinusitis, sore throat, nonproductive cough, sneeze, headache, malaise, chills, low-grade fever, laryngitis, and arthralgia.[8,9] The number of coughs, sneezes, and times blowing the nose per day can be used to track progression of URI since occurrence of these events decreases as recovery occurs.[9]

URI is contagious, spreading from person to person through respiratory secretions.[8] Hand-to-hand contact after touching the mouth, nose, or eyes appears to be the most efficient mode of transmission.[9] The virus is active for at least 8 days following the initial infection, during which the person may transmit the virus, although communicability is highest in the first 72 hours.[9,10] Frequent hand washing and avoidance of infected persons can prevent the spread of URI.

Recognition of URI and support of the immune system with rest, fluids, and nutrition can limit the duration of the infection. Athletes who are experiencing symptoms of URI should limit their activities at least until the fever resolves to avoid fatigue and dehydration, as well as to prevent infecting teammates.[8,9] If no evidence of cardiac, pulmonary, gastrointestinal, or other systemic involvement appears, full activity can resume within a few days.[4,5,8,10] Table 10-4 provides general guidelines for managing suspected URI in athletes.

Influenza (Flu)

"Flu" is often incorrectly used as a general term for URI but actually describes a disease caused by a specific virus. Influenza outbreaks occur annually, usually in the fall and winter months. Influenza virus mutates slightly each year, rendering vaccination (injection of deactivated virus antigens, to stimulate antibody formation) only partially effective. Influenza virus spreads easily through respiratory secretions, either by inhaling airborne droplets or by touching contaminated objects. After incubation (time between infection and appearance of symptoms) of 2 days, fever, myalgia, headache, and URI symptoms appear.[11] As infection progresses, a productive cough (ie, cough with sputum, signifying lower respiratory infection) develops, as well as pharyngitis, conjunctivitis, and nausea.

The active stage lasts 2 to 3 days, followed by a reduction in fever, and the appearance of diaphoresis and fatigue (ie, "breaking" fever) that may last several additional days. Secondary infections of the respiratory tract with additional bacteria or viruses may coexist, producing hemoptysis, recurrent fever, purulent sputum, or progressive dyspnea. Rarely, Reye's syndrome (signaled by altered mental status and severe vomiting) occurs in children with influenza (or other viral infection) who have ingested aspirin. Aspirin is therefore not generally recommended for use among children.

Pneumonia and Tuberculosis: Typical Bacterial Respiratory Infections

A variety of bacteria may colonize the respiratory system and cause a number of diseases. Two of the most common are pneumonia, caused primarily by streptococcal or staphylococcal bacteria, and pulmonary tuberculosis, caused by mycobacteria.

Table 10-4

MANAGEMENT OF URI IN ATHLETES

Associated Symptoms	Action
Rhinorrhea, rhinitis, sinusitis, sore throat, nonproductive cough, sneezing	Allow to begin exercise; if symptoms clear, continue exercise as tolerated; if symptoms worsen, stop exercise
Fever, productive cough, myalgia, vomiting, or diarrhea	Do not workout for 10 to 14 days and refer to physician

Persons with chronic medical illnesses, respiratory diseases, long-term hospitalization, or a compromised immune system are at increased risk for pneumonia. Streptococcal or staphylococcal bacteria, fairly common in the nasopharynx and upper respiratory tract, invade lung tissue when immune function is suppressed. High fever, cough with purulent sputum, hyperpnea, crackles upon auscultation, and pleuritic pain occur after infection. Pneumonia is treated with antibiotics specific to the invading bacteria. Oxygen supplementation may be required if pulmonary compromise is severe. Among elderly or severely ill persons, pneumonia can be fatal.

Pulmonary tuberculosis (TB), in contrast, may be asymptomatic for long periods. Vague, nondisabling symptoms (eg, slight fatigue, malaise) may occur, but a persistent cough is commonly the first symptom. As the disease progressively destroys lung tissue, hemoptysis or spontaneous pneumothorax may occur (see Chapter Four). Patches of atelectasis cause absent breath sounds upon auscultation of the affected regions. General pulmonary edema may also occur, causing decreased auscultated breath sounds. Diagnosis is made with x-rays and laboratory tests.

To be effective, pharmacological TB treatment must be early, organism-specific, and complete. TB is extremely contagious, so a person known to have TB infection must be isolated from others. Using strict precautions, including gloves, face mask, face shield, and protective gowning, prevents exposure to the respiratory secretions of a person with TB.

Infective Myocarditis

Infective myocarditis, although uncommon, is caused by relatively common organisms. Coxsackieviruses, which usually cause GI symptoms, are encountered by most people throughout life.[3,12-16] Some respiratory viruses can also cause myocarditis, as can bacteria such as streptococcus.[17]

In general, known infection with Coxsackie, streptococcal virus, or an active URI should lead to the prohibition of athletic participation.[3] Gradual deterioration in physical performance may indicate secondary or subacute myocarditis but occurs in less than half of such cases.[3] In known infectious myocarditis, vigorous activity should be avoided for at least 2 months after resolution of acute symptoms and resumed only under the advice of a physician.[3,15,16]

Gastrointestinal Infections

Gastrointestinal (GI) infections include viral gastroenteritis, food poisoning, and "traveler's" diarrhea.[8] Viral gastroenteritis ("stomach flu") causes severe vomiting, diarrhea, and abdominal spasms, and is accompanied by fever and myalgia.[8,18] The virus is contracted by ingesting matter contaminated by feces, known as the "fecal-oral" route of transmission, most commonly a result of improper hand washing by food preparers. The syndrome, which lasts a few days, is usually self-limiting and rarely life-threatening in healthy young people.[8] Primary interventions include rest and maintaining hydration.[8,18] Occasionally, hydration by intravenous fluids is required. Antidiarrheal and antiemetic (inhibit vomiting) medications are not recommended since they delay elimination of the virus.[8] Return to participation usually occurs within a week, depending on resolution of symptoms and hydration status.

Food poisoning occurs with ingestion of foodborne bacteria, most commonly staphylococcus.[8] The bacteria, usually from the hands or respiratory secretions of a food handler, produces a toxin as it multiplies on unrefrigerated meat or dairy products.[8] Within a couple of hours of ingestion, severe vomiting and diarrhea occur and persist for several hours. Hydration is usually the only treatment necessary. Again, antiemetic and antidiarrheal drugs are not recommended since they delay elimination of the bacteria.[8]

Traveler's diarrhea is so named since infectious diarrhea frequently occurs in persons from the United States while traveling to foreign (particularly Asian and South American) countries. Bacteria (E. coli, salmonella, etc.) or viruses are transmitted through the fecal-oral route from improper hand washing, poor handling of uncooked food, improperly cooked food, and contamination of public water sources. This syndrome is similar to other GI infections, including diarrhea, abdominal spasms, and fatigue (from dehydration and decreased caloric intake) that lasts up to 3 days.[8] Avoidance of potentially contaminated foods and water (ie, consume only bottled fluids and packaged foods) and consumption of prophylactic bismuth sub-susalicylate (eg, Pepto-Bismol) every 6 hours throughout travel can prevent infection while traveling. Treatment is similar to viral gastroenteritis and food poisoning, involving primarily rest and hydration. Antidiarrheal medications can be used with traveler's diarrhea unless fever (indicating gastroenteritis) or bloody stool (hematochezia) occurs.[8]

Urinary Tract Infections

Urinary tract infection (UTI) by bacteria, fungi, or parasites are very common. Bacterial infections are by far the most prevalent UTI. Regardless of invading organism, possible consequences include urethritis (inflamed urethra), cystitis (inflamed bladder), prostatitis (inflamed prostate), and pyelonephritis (inflamed kidney) as the organism progresses up the urinary tract. Symptomatic infection with yeast (candida albicans), causing vulvular irritation, is very common in women, although men can carry and transmit yeast infections without experiencing symptoms themselves. Signs and symptoms of UTI depend on the primary site of colonization in the urinary tract (Table 10-5). Treatment consists of antibiotics or antifungal medications, as well as analgesics or antipruritics (inhibit itching) to control symptoms.

Sexually Transmitted Diseases

Sexually transmitted diseases (STDs) are communicated to sexual partners by direct contact with genital wounds or body fluids. These diseases can infect the rectum, eyes, and mouth in addition to the genitals. Use of condoms reduces the risk of contracting an STD,

Table 10-5

SIGNS AND SYMPTOMS OF URINARY TRACT INFECTION BY SITE OF COLONIZATION

Site	Signs and Symptoms
Urethra	Dysuria, discharge
Bladder	Dysuria, urgency, decreased urine volume, nocturia, back pain, pyuria or hematuria
Prostate	Fever, urgency, back pain, dysuria, nocturia, hematuria
Kidney	Fever, back pain, vomiting, costovertebral tenderness

although they do not guarantee prevention. Contact of any mucous membrane with contaminated fluids or lesions greatly increases the probability of infection.

Gonorrhea

Bacteria that cause gonorrhea incubate for 1 to 3 weeks, then induce purulent urethral discharge and painful dysuria. Other mucous membranes (mouth, throat, eyes, rectum) may be infected, producing pain, erythema, edema, or purulent exudate. A significant portion of infected persons, however, experience no symptoms but remain contagious and can transmit the organism to others. Gonorrhea often coexists with other STDs, such as chlamydia and syphilis (see below). Vigorous and meticulous medical care is necessary to address gonorrhea and all comorbid infections. Sexual contact with others must be strictly avoided until the infection is eliminated. Recent (previous 3 to 6 months) sexual partners should be contacted, examined, and treated if necessary.

Chlamydia

Chlamydia, estimated to be the most common STD, is a bacterial infection with an incubation period of 1 to 4 weeks in men. Infected women, although usually asymptomatic, transmit the bacteria to their sexual partners. Symptoms include painful dysuria and clear or purulent urethral discharge. Similar to gonorrhea, other mucous membranes may be affected. Treatment is by antibiotics and screening for comorbid STDs. Abstention from sexual activity is required until infection resolves. Recent (3 to 6 months) sexual partners should be contacted, examined, and treated.

Syphilis

Syphilis is another bacteria that invades the urogenital system during sexual contact, although the organism ultimately infects other systems, including the nervous and cardiovascular systems. Symptoms may not occur for up to 3 months after initial exposure. However, a painless epithelial lesion on the region exposed to the bacteria, called a chancre, appears and spontaneously resolves within 2 months. Inguinal lymphadenitis may occur but are usually not tender and may not be noticed. A skin rash erupts within 2 months and may persist for 2 to 3 additional months. Low-grade fever, fatigue, headache, loss of appetite, and myalgia may also appear during this stage.

If untreated, the disease goes into remission, sometimes for decades. Invasion of bone, skin, myocardium, or the central nervous system eventually occurs, leading to serious and irreversible changes in those systems. Cardiac and central nervous system complications are the most severe, disabling, and ultimately fatal. Treatment begins with early recognition and consists of appropriate antibiotic therapy and identification of a coexisting STD.

Genital Warts

Various papillomaviruses cause genital warts. External warts, cauliflower-like in appearance, appear on the genitals 1 to 6 months after infection. Internal warts may appear on the rectum, vagina, or cervix, requiring physical examination by a physician to identify them. Treatment is by surgical removal and topical medications, although recurrences are common and, in some cases, total resolution may not be possible. During exacerbation, sexual abstinence is required to prevent communicating the virus. Some papillomaviruses have been implicated as causes of cervical cancer.

Herpes

Genital herpes, caused by the herpes simplex virus, occurs after contact with the genital lesions of an infected person. Herpes can affect any mucous membrane, most commonly the genitals. Once infected, the virus invades and remains in the ganglia of the associated nerves for the remainder of the host's lifetime. Periodically, the virus reactivates and causes recurrence of the lesions.

Small vesicles appear within a week of initial infection. These lesions are circular, painful, appear in clusters, and generally heal in 1 to 2 weeks. Dysuria, paresthesia, and other neurological signs may appear. General systemic signs, including fever, malaise, and inguinal lymphadenitis, may present after initial infection. Subsequent occurrences usually have shorter duration and are less symptomatic. Diagnosis requires medical laboratory tests. Treatment involves medications to control symptoms during outbreaks and limit recurrent episodes. Abstention from sexual activity when lesions are present is essential.

Pelvic Inflammatory Disease

Pelvic inflammatory disease (PID) results from infection of the cervix, uterus, or fallopian tubes. Chlamydia and gonorrhea bacteria, usually contracted during sexual intercourse, are the most common organisms invading these organs. Signs and symptoms include abdominal pain, high-grade fever, nausea, and purulent or bloody vaginal discharge. PID can cause infertility, ectopic pregnancies, chronic pelvic pain, or death if untreated. Once the organism is identified, immediate antibiotic treatment begins. Clinically, signs and symptoms of acute PID are difficult to discern from ectopic pregnancy (see Chapter Seven), thus requiring emergency medical examination.

Neurological Infections

Bacteria and viruses can invade the CNS and cause inflammation of the meninges, called meningitis. These organisms enter the CNS through the bloodstream, cranial sinuses, or after surgical or traumatic wounds that expose the meninges. The CNS has relatively few immune defenses, so bacteria replicates rapidly. As the concentration of bacteria increases, fluid is drawn into the cranium and cranial blood vessels. Intracranial pressure increases rapidly, causing neurological compression and ischemia. In addition, the inflammatory response alters the permeability of the blood-brain barrier, allowing inappropriate substances into the brain and further increasing pressure. Blood pressure drops rapidly and death may occur from shock or cerebral ischemia.

Bacterial meningitis caused by streptococcus or meningococcus bacteria can be fatal within hours of infection. An intolerable headache, very rigid neck, violent vomiting, and rapidly rising fever occur and worsen over a few hours. Altered cognition, syncope, seizures, and coma may also occur. Clinical signs include a rash on the head and inability to flex the neck passively without hip and knee flexion, known as Brudzinski's sign (see Chapter Eight). Emergency transport for aggressive antibiotic therapy is the course of treatment.

Other organisms, including viruses, drugs, lead poisoning, and parasites, can cause less severe forms of meningitis. Differentiation, however, often requires medical procedures and laboratory tests performed by a physician. When presented with a history, symptoms, and signs consistent with meningitis, the athletic trainer should document vital signs (particularly body temperature) and make an emergency medical referral.

Musculoskeletal Infections

Osteomyelitis is a term that describes bone infection. Usually osteomyelitis occurs when an infection in surrounding tissue is transmitted to the bone. Open fractures, recent orthopedic surgery, and prosthetic joints increase risk of osteomyelitis. Once a bone is infected, blood supply becomes compromised, increasing necrosis and infection in surrounding bone. Signs and symptoms include fever, weight loss, fatigue, and inflammation in the affected area. Definitive diagnosis usually requires x-rays or other imaging studies with biopsy (surgical tissue harvesting) to identify the organism. Antibiotic therapy, surgical debridement, and bone grafting may be necessary to halt progression of the disease.

Septic arthrosis is the infection of a joint, which may result in destruction of synovium and cartilage, called septic arthritis. Immunocompromise or malnutrition increases risk of septic arthrosis. The organism invades the joint through wounds, the bloodstream, or surrounding tissues. The athletic trainer may encounter this condition among persons who have had recent orthopedic surgery or deep subcutaneous wound. Rapid inflammation of the joint occurs well beyond normal postoperative inflammatory response, and extreme pain and intolerance of joint movement may appear. Fever may not occur if the infection is limited to one joint. Medical referral for diagnosis and antibiotic treatment is appropriate.

Rheumatoid Arthritis

Rheumatoid arthritis (RA), a chronic condition characterized by progressive degeneration of multiple joints, occurs when the immune system perceives the synovium as a foreign tissue and attacks it. Bilateral inflammation of several joints, particularly the hands, feet, and ankles, and morning stiffness lasting 30 to 60 minutes are early indicators. As RA progresses, joint deformities, ruptured tendons, and disability develop. Persons with RA require lifetime medications and may undergo reconstructive surgery. Precautions, such as avoiding high joint loads and extreme ranges of motion, are required.

Juvenile RA occurs among adolescents with a clinical presentation similar to adult RA, although the prognosis is considerably better. Nonsteroidal anti-inflammatory drugs and occasionally corticosteroids are prescribed to limit synovial inflammation. Participation in athletics should be under the guidance of the treating physician and depends on severity of the disease.

Chronic Fatigue and Overtraining Syndrome

Overtraining (excessive athletic conditioning without adequate recovery) may result in behavioral and physical changes. Increases in cortisol in response to chronic physical stress impair the ability to respond to hypoglycemia during and after exercise and suppresses the immune system.[19] This produces irritability, apathy, unusual fatigue, declining performance, loss of appetite, excessive thirst, and insomnia.[19,20] In addition, certain physical signs such as increased resting heart rate, blood pressure, body temperature, or changes in body weight or bowel habits may occur.[20] Rest and change in training routine is the definitive treatment.

General Contagious Diseases

Infectious Mononucleosis (Mono)

Caused by the Epstein-Barr virus (EBV), which is a variant of the herpes virus carried in saliva, mono is common among persons age 15 to 25 years.[5,8] Repeated and prolonged exposure is required to induce infection, although an estimated 90% of Americans over age 30 show antibodies to EBV, thus indicating previous infection.[8,17]

Mono follows a typical course. The incubation period lasts over a month and is followed by 3 to 5 days of headache, fatigue, loss of appetite, and myalgia.[5,17] The following 1 or 2 weeks present a severe sore throat, enlargement of the tonsils, moderate fever, bilateral cervical lymphadenopathy, small red spots on the soft palate, splenomegaly in over half of all cases, and hepatomegaly in about one-third of all cases.[5,8,17] Treatment for mono consists of rest, hydration, analgesics, and antipyretics (to inhibit fever).[8] Rarely, corticosteroids are prescribed for symptomatic relief but do not decrease duration of the infection.[8] Antibiotics are not indicated unless a bacterial infection occurs.

Although signs and symptoms rarely persist more than a month, athletic performance may be impaired for up to 3 months.[8] Mono causes splenomegaly, predisposing the spleen to rupture, primarily in males within the first 3 weeks of symptoms.[5,8] Thus, to protect the spleen, a minimum of 3 weeks after onset of clinical symptoms should pass before allowing return to athletics.[8] A physician should make the decision to allow return to participation, which depends largely on spleen size, absence of fever, resolution of symptoms, and normal medical liver tests. Return to full participation takes an additional 1 to 2 weeks and is usually limited by fatigue.[8]

Human Immunodeficiency Virus and Acquired Immunodeficiency Syndrome

Although no confirmed cases of human immunodeficiency virus (HIV) transmission have occurred in sports (two unconfirmed cases have been reported),[4] it is hypothetically possible to contract the virus through fist-fighting or other violent physical contact.[2] Hence, athletic trainers should follow standard precautions (gloves, avoid contact with body fluids) to avoid exposure to blood or other body fluids. HIV has been documented among health care workers after exposure to body fluids of infected persons. Most cases, however, are contracted through sexual contact or sharing of intravenous needles.

HIV primarily impairs T-cells but also affects B-cells, phagocytes, and other immune system cells, thus impairing both the specific and general aspects of the cell-mediated component of the immune system. In addition, the humoral aspect of immunity is also impaired since the B-cells, which mediate protein complement and immunoglobin (antibody) function, are affected. The medical result is suppression of the immune system, which increases the risk of multiple infections.

Initial signs and symptoms, which appear within a month of HIV infection, include fever, arthralgia, skin rash, and lymphadenitis throughout the body. These, which may be mistaken for influenza or other viral infections, persist for 1 to 3 weeks, then subside. The person can communicate HIV during this asymptomatic stage. Without treatment, neurological, hematological, gastrointestinal, dermatological, and pulmonary infections appear within 3 to 10 years. The presence of certain infections as a result of HIV infection constitute a syndrome called acquired immunodeficiency syndrome (AIDS). About half of persons infected with HIV develop AIDS within 10 years.

Treatment of initial HIV infection includes a complex regimen of antiviral agents, which inhibit HIV replication and delays onset of AIDS. AIDS, once developed, is also treated with antiviral medications. Other treatments are provided depending on which comorbid infections are present. Exercise among persons with HIV slows progression of infection and improves physical ability.[4] Currently, no cure exists for HIV infection or AIDS. HIV remains contagious regardless of antiviral therapy. Strictly avoiding contact with body fluids prevents communication of HIV.

Hepatitis B Virus

Hepatitis B virus (HBV) is more common, present in more body tissues and fluids, active outside the body for a longer time, and more easily communicated than HIV. Fortunately, standard precautions prevent infection by HBV.[21] To date, the United States has no reported cases of HBV transmission during sports, although it has occurred in other countries.[2] Vaccination against HBV is available. Health care workers should undergo the 6-month series of three injections to decrease risk of contracting HBV.[21] Chapter Five reviews the signs, symptoms, and treatment of hepatitis.

Ear, Eye, Nose, and Throat Infections

These structures provide the primary boundaries between the internal organs and the external environment. Unfortunately, their warm and moist environment also provides ideal conditions to develop infection. Thus, because of high exposure and fertile environment, infections in these areas are very common. Lab Activity 8 outlines the use of an otoscope to examine the ears and nose.[22,23]

Otitis Externa

Frequent exposure to water (eg, swimmers) flushes the protective cerumen (wax) from the ear and can cause infections of the external ear canal called *otitis externa*.[8,17,24] The constant moisture also softens the ear canal tissue, providing opportunity for infection by bacteria or fungi.[8] Lakes, rivers, or improperly chlorinated pools commonly contain bacteria responsible for these infections. Using cotton swabs to scour the ear can further irritate the canal, thus increasing risk of infection.

Otitis externa produces ear drainage, canal swelling, and erythema (which can be visualized by otoscope).[22,23] These effects decrease hearing, cause itching, and produce pain when the auricle is gently pulled.[8,17] Treatment involves irrigation with sterile saline or hydrogen peroxide, inserting antibiotic or antifungal ear drops, and avoiding immersion.[8,17,24] Usually within 3 days, pain and erythema decrease and swimming can be resumed.[8] Using ear plugs while swimming, carefully drying the ears, using drying agents (eg, boric acid solution), and avoiding the use of swabs are some simple protective measures.[8]

Impacted Cerumen

Impacted cerumen can cause symptoms similar to otitis externa, including itching, pain, and impaired hearing. A physician may remove the cerumen by scraping with a blunt tool (under direct visualization) or suctioning the ear canal. Irrigation with saline or other solutions is not recommended if a history of ear infection or drainage exists. Self-application of cotton swabs or solvents to remove the cerumen may irritate the skin, creating opportunity for infection to develop, and should be avoided.[23]

Conjunctivitis

Conjunctivitis denotes inflammation of the lining of the posterior eyelid and eyeball margins (the conjunctiva). Inflammation can result from allergens or infection by bacteria or viruses.[24] Burning (infection) or itching (allergy) with purulent (infection) or mucoid (allergy) drainage from the eye occurs. The "white" of the eyeball appears swollen and red, leading to the layman's term "pink eye." Allergic reactions usually affect both eyes, whereas an infection begins unilaterally. Infectious conjunctivitis, however, spreads quickly to the opposite eye, usually after rubbing first the infected eye and then the other.

Treatment of infectious conjunctivitis is with antibiotic eyedrops or oral medications. The person must be instructed to avoid rubbing the face and to practice meticulous hand washing to avoid spreading the disease. Allergic conjunctivitis is usually treated with antihistamines or anti-inflammatories. Medical referral for definitive diagnosis and treatment is indicated.

Stye

Infection of an eyelid duct or follicle is called a stye.[24] Caused most often by staphylococcal bacteria, the stye produces localized pain on the margin of the eyelid. Lacrimation (producing tears) and a sensation of "something in the eye" also occur. Inspection by gently rolling back the eyelid with a cotton swab reveals a round, red lump on the margin. A stye can be treated with warm, wet compresses for 10 minutes a few times a day and should completely resolve in a few days. Lesions observed in other parts of the eyelid or eye require prompt referral to an ophthalmologist.

Eye Pain

Very severe eye pain accompanied by systemic symptoms (eg, nausea) or significant changes in vision (ie, severe photophobia or blurring, partial loss of visual field) suggest serious pathology, such as acute glaucoma (increased pressure in the eye). In such situations, a risk of permanent vision loss exists. Emergency medical care is indicated.

Infective Laryngitis, Pharyngitis, Tonsillitis

Infection and inflammation of the throat are common symptoms of other immune system pathology (eg, URI, STD, allergies), although they can occur as isolated conditions. The pharynx consists of the most posterior part of the oral cavity and superior part of the throat. The larynx, or "voice box," contains the vocal cords and lies inferior to the pharynx in the throat. The tonsils are small glands that reside in the lateral pharynx. Numerous infectious organisms can invade these structures.

Pharyngitis and tonsillitis both produce throat pain, painful or difficult swallowing (and subsequent avoidance of food), and pain in the ears when swallowing. Inspection reveals a red (erythematous) throat with purulent or mucoid exudate covering the pharynx (pharyngitis) or notably inflamed tonsils (tonsillitis). Laryngitis causes changes in the quality of the voice, such as hoarseness or complete inability to speak. Itching may require frequent throat

Table 10-6

COMMON SKIN LESIONS ASSOCIATED WITH INFECTIONS AND ALLERGIC REACTIONS

Lesion	Description	Examples
Vesicle	Subcutaneous accumulations of serous fluid < 5 mm	Impetigo, herpes simplex
Bulla	Subcutaneous accumulations of serous fluid > 5 mm	Blister
Papule	Small epidermal tumors	Wart, skin cancer
Pustule	Subcutaneous accumulations of pus	Acne, furuncles
Wheal	Circumscribed regions of inflamed skin	Hives
Scales	Excess epidermis forming small flakes	Late-stage tinea pedis

clearing. Fever, difficulty or pain with swallowing, or even dyspnea may occur with severe laryngitis. A physician may observe purulent exudate on the larynx with a laryngoscope.

After a physician rules out serious pathology, treatment for throat infection is rest, analgesics, and nutrition. Contagious bacterial infections, such as streptococcal pharyngitis (strep throat), may require antibiotics and temporary isolation (24 to 36 hours) to prevent communicating the infectious organism to others.

Skin Infections

Very common among athletes, skin infections can be viral, bacterial, or fungal. Effects of environmental heat and moisture, profuse sweating, frequent skin trauma, and tight-fitting athletic equipment combine to predispose the skin to infection.[2,4] Table 10-6 gives various lesions associated with skin infections.

Bacterial Skin Infections

The skin may be invaded by staphylococcal or streptococcal bacteria.[2,4,24] Most bacterial skin infections colonize hair follicles, are highly contagious, and are transmitted by direct contact. These infections require bandaging, avoiding the sharing of equipment and towels, and meticulous personal hygiene to prevent spread to team members or competitors.

Treatment primarily depends on the extent of the lesion. A small lesion may resolve quickly with basic wound care (ie, keep the area clean and dry, avoid irritations such as friction, and cover for protection and to contain wound drainage). Larger, deeper infections, however, may require topical or oral antibiotics and incision (lancing) by a physician to drain the wound. Rarely, bacterial skin infections, particularly from carbuncles, spread through the blood to other organs unless properly managed.[2,8] Table 10-7 outlines general treatment for various bacterial skin lesions.[2,8,24]

Table 10-7

TREATMENT OF BACTERIAL SKIN LESIONS

Acne vulgaris	Clean frequently with antibiotic soap, application of topical drying agents, wash bed linens and helmet straps frequently, possibly ultraviolet or hormonal therapies.
Folliculitis	Clean with antibiotic soap, topical and oral antibiotics (7 to 10 days).
Furunculosis/boils	Clean skin frequently with antibiotic soap, warm compresses, oral antibiotics; physician may lance boil if distended with fluid.
Carbuncles	Same as for furuncle.
Impetigo	Antibiotic soap or hydrogen peroxide debridement of crust, topical antibiotic.

Fungal Skin Infections

Fungal skin infections (tinea) invade many regions of the body, including the feet (tinea pedis or athlete's foot), the groin (tinea cruris or jock itch), and other areas (tinea corporis or ringworm and tinea versicolor).[8,24] Fungal growth is exacerbated by heat, moisture, and lack of light, often inhabiting body parts constantly enclosed in clothes or shoes. Fungi are highly contagious and can be spread by direct contact with infected skin or by contact with contaminated surfaces.[8]

Tinea pedis and tinea cruris produce scaly or blistered skin, erythema, itching, burning, and occasionally serous (translucent) drainage.[8] Tinea corporis appears as red rings with clear centers in the skin. Tinea versicolor produces irregular patches of depigmented, white, scaly skin. Fungal infections also occur in the toenails (called onychomycosis), causing discoloration, deformity, detachment, and thickening.

Treatment of fungal skin infections include topical medications and preventative behaviors such as alternating pairs of shoes or workout clothing to allow drying, using clean cotton clothing and powders to absorb moisture, showering frequently, and avoiding contact with potentially contaminated surfaces (eg, shower floors).[24] Tinea infections resolve within 2 weeks with appropriate care.[8] Repigmentation after tinea versicolor may take 2 months.[8] Onychomycosis can persist for weeks or months.

Viral Skin Infections

Viral skin infections include warts (verrucae) and herpes simplex.[4,8] Papillomaviruses cause both common (verrucae plana) and plantar (verrucae plantaris) warts. Common warts usually appear on the hands as irregular, rough bumps.[8] Plantar warts occur on the weightbearing surfaces of the feet, appearing as small, thick spots of skin that actually extend deep into the skin. Plantar warts produce pinpoint bleeding when trimmed, unlike calluses.[8]

Papillomaviruses incubate about 6 months before producing a wart and can be contracted by direct contact or contaminated surfaces or clothing.[8] Once contracted, warts are notoriously hard to eliminate. Common warts, primarily a cosmetic concern, can be removed surgically or with topical medications. Plantar warts can be very painful and may inhibit performance. Treatment of plantar warts involves regular application of topical plasters of salicylic acid.[24]

Herpes simplex virus can affect the face (cold sores, fever blisters, or herpes labialis) or hands and spreads through direct contact. Lesions appear as small fluid-filled vesicles surrounded by erythematous skin. The vesicles erupt and form a crust within 3 days of appearing. This crust persists for up to a week and may be accompanied by general systemic symptoms (fever, myalgia, headache, etc).[4,8] Physical or psychological stress (trauma, illness, menstruation) can produce recurrences of the lesions.[8,24] Athletes with active lesions should be withheld from participation to prevent spread to other athletes.[4] No cure currently exists, although viral-inhibiting medications may be prescribed.

A member of the herpes simplex virus family produces herpes gladitorium, which is similar to other herpes simplex skin infections, but appears on large, flat skin surfaces (arms, legs, back).[2,24] Lesions usually heal in a few days, but herpes gladitorium is highly infectious when vesicles are present. The virus can spread to the eyes or other mucous membranes and recurs only occasionally.[2] Herpes gladitorium is usually self-limiting, requiring only removal from competition for a few days, avoidance of irritation of the region, and appropriate wound care.[2,24]

Molluscum Contagiosum

Molluscum contagiosum is a virus that appears on the hands, arms, or face as firm, raised lesions, often near an abrasion or laceration in the skin. Transmission occurs by direct contact. Treatment involves surgical incision and cautery with electricity or liquid nitrogen.[8,24] Following healing of the surgical wound, participation can be resumed immediately.

Anaerobic Skin Infections

Wound infections with anaerobic clostridium bacteria cause tetanus and gas gangrene, both of which are potentially fatal.[25] Their spores often remain dormant for years until introduction to an anaerobic (without oxygen) biological environment. A penetrating wound (including use of contaminated syringes), crush injury, or open fracture may provide this type of environment.

With tetanus, systemic signs appear a few days after exposure (eg, fever, myalgia, headache). Severe rigidity of the jaw, neck, back, and abdominal muscles develop rapidly, and painful spasms occur with small perturbations or vibrations.[25] Asphyxia can occur when pharyngeal muscles spasm. Preventative immunization in the United States begins in infancy and is repeated every 5 to 7 years. A penetrating wound in a person who has not been recently inoculated requires appropriate wound management (ie, cleaning, irrigation, debridement) and an immediate tetanus booster.[25] Fully developed tetanus requires medical life support and antitoxin therapy.

Gas gangrene occurs within hours of infection as anaerobic bacteria destroy muscle and connective tissue, producing large volumes of subcutaneous gas. Severe pain and swelling appear, and the limb turns deep red and progresses quickly to black.[25] Without extensive, immediate emergency surgical limb debridement, shock, and death result. The organism for gas gangrene reproduces in the GI tract (among other places) of animals, thus necessitating the avoidance of pastures as practice fields.

Fortunately, both tetanus and gas gangrene are relatively rare, usually occurring with severe or deep penetrating wounds. Prompt medical referral of such wounds, particularly when tetanus booster status is uncertain, and close communication with the treating physician is appropriate.

Table 10-8
PREVENTING INFECTIOUS DISEASES

- Appropriate diet, recovery time between workouts, and sleep.
- Individual water bottles, towels, uniforms, and personal equipment.
- Individual dose packaging for ointments and topical medications.
- Immediate showering after participation.
- Frequent laundering of uniforms.
- Recognition, proper care, and protection of infectious skin lesions.
- Vaccination of athletes and health care workers against preventable diseases (measles, mumps, rubella, DPT, influenza, HBV, etc).
- Prompt cleaning and covering of open wounds and body-fluid saturated uniforms.
- Disinfecting soiled surfaces or equipment promptly.
- Personal protective equipment and strict enforcement of hand washing and standard precautions protocols for medical and laundry personnel.
- Immunization (particularly tetanus, measles, and childhood vaccinations) should be current; may need to update immunizations when traveling to specific regions or countries.
- Avoid exertion and contact with teammates during active infection.
- Avoid possibly contaminated water (lakes, rivers).
- Meticulous environmental control of public areas (showers, swimming pools, etc).

Prevention of Infectious Disease

Table 10-8 provides general guidelines for the prevention of infectious diseases in athletic and health care environments.[2,4,8,21,26] Position statements of various medical associations and reviews regulations for health care facilities regarding control of infectious disease are available.[26-28]

Allergic Reactions and Anaphylaxis

An allergy is a localized, cell-mediated immune reaction following exposure to a substance perceived by the body as toxic (an antigen), including certain foods, pollens, molds, and insect bites. Release of histamine and other vasodilatory and inflammatory chemical mediators from mast cells produce this reaction. Generalized allergic skin reactions are called urticaria, producing wheals (hives) that itch and may or may not drain. Mechanical, psychogenic, or physical agents can also produce urticaria.

Anaphylaxis is a systemic, massive allergic response, including smooth muscle contraction and widespread vasodilation that produces shock. Rarely and with unknown etiology, anaphylaxis induced by physical activity (exercise-induced anaphylaxis) can cause death. Anaphylaxis can also occur following exposure to specific antigens, most commonly insect bites, in hypersensitive persons. Avoidance of known physical triggers or allergens constitutes primary prevention. Emergency treatment to counter the histamine response, such as injectable epinephrine, may be necessary in extreme reactions. History of known allergens and reactions should be obtained during the preparticipation examination and a plan of care developed to manage accidental exposures. Athletes with known anaphylactic reactions should have epinephrine available while participating in activities where exposure is possible.

PEDIATRIC CONCERNS

Childhood Infectious Diseases

Chicken pox (varicella virus), mumps (paramyxovirus), and measles (rubeola) are common among children, but can be contracted at any age. These conditions spread rapidly through day care centers and schools. Close physical proximity and contact, insulated environments, and sharing of food utensils and toys between children contribute to such outbreaks. While relatively harmless in otherwise healthy children, these diseases can cause severe complications among children with immunosuppression and susceptible (ie, not previously infected) adults. Thus, controlling spread of these diseases is important.

Chicken Pox

Chicken pox (varicella virus) incubates approximately 2 weeks, then causes general systemic symptoms (low-grade fever, fatigue, headache) and widespread skin vesicles that erupt, itch, and drain. The virus is most contagious immediately preceding and during vesicle formation. Chicken pox often causes epidemics in schools or other children's peer groups (eg, sports teams). Once vesicles burst, drain, and crust, the virus is no longer contagious.

Mumps

Mumps (a paramyxovirus) incubates 2 to 4 weeks, then causes general systemic signs and symptoms shortly before salivary and parotid glands begin to swell. This bilateral swelling causes a characteristic swollen (chipmunk) face. Additional signs and symptoms include dysphagia, high-grade fever, and tenderness in the swollen glands. The virus is contagious (less so than chicken pox or measles) from about a week before glandular swelling through resolution.

Measles

Measles (rubeola, also a paramyxovirus) incubates about 2 weeks, then initiates a flu-like syndrome (fever, myalgia, malaise) followed within a week by numerous, characteristic red skin eruptions. High-grade fever (over 104°F) develops and lasts several days, after which the condition resolves. Measles is contagious from the time of infection until the rash subsides.

Immunization

Infection with these viruses usually ensures lifetime immunity. Standard pediatric immunizations include mumps and measles vaccination. More recently, chicken pox vaccines have been developed, but are administered only to persons at increased risk to exposure or severe complications.

SUMMARY

Infection is invasion of a tissue or organ by colonies of organisms, such as bacteria, viruses, parasites, or fungi. The immune system combats infection by using both general and organism-specific mechanisms. Thus, infection produces signs and symptoms that are both general, including fever, myalgia, malaise, and fatigue, and specific to the affected organ or system. Contagious diseases are extremely common and affect physical performance. The majority of these conditions can be treated with rest and support of the immune system, although some require antibiotic medications or other medical care. Following relatively simple procedures can significantly reduce the risk of spreading most infectious diseases.

RESOURCES

Dermatology

- atlife.com dermatology site. www.atdermatology.com/dermatology
- Yahoo directory. dir.yahoo.com/Health/Diseases_and_Conditions/Skin_Conditions

Dermatology Images

- Emedicine.com, choose a dermatological condition, then click on the tab labeled "Pictures" near the top of the screen. www.emedicine.com/derm/contents.htm
- Medi-smart.com index page containing links to pages that contain images. medi-smart.com/derm2.htm
- National Skin Center page contains descriptions and images of over 75 common skin disorders. www.nsc.gov.sg/commskin/skin.html
- University of Iowa Department of Dermatology. tray.dermatology.uiowa.edu/DPT/Path-Index.htm

Immunology

- atlife.com allergy and infectious disease sites:

  www.atallergy.com/allergy

  www.atinfections.com/id
- Yahoo directory. dir.yahoo.com/Health/Diseases_and_Conditions/Infectious_Diseases

Infection Control Guidelines from the Centers for Disease Control and Prevention

- Development of Isolation Precautions Guidelines outlines the differences between "Universal Precautions" and "Standard Precautions." www.cdc.gov/ncidod/hip/isolat/isopart1.htm
- Guidelines for Isolation Precautions in Hospitals (table of contents). www.cdc.gov/ncidod/hip/isolat/isolat.htm
- Standard Precautions types of isolation used in health care facilities. www.cdc.gov/ncidod/hip/isolat/isopart2.htm

REFERENCES

1. Pyne DB, Gleeson M. Effects of intensive exercise training on immunity in athletes. *Int J Sports Med.* 1998;19(Suppl):S183-S194.

2. Mast EE, Goodman RA. Prevention of infectious disease transmission in sports. *Sports Med.* 1997;24(1):1-7.

3. Friman G, Ilbäck NG. Acute infection: metabolic responses, effects on performance, interaction with exercise, and myocarditis. *Int J Sports Med.* 1998;19:S172-S182.

4. Brenner IKM, Shek PN, Shephard RJ. Infection in athletes. *Sports Med.* 1994;17(2):86-107.

5. Roberts JA. Viral illnesses and sports performance. *Sports Med.* 1986;3:296-303.

6. Nieman DC. Risk of upper respiratory tract infection in athletes: an epidemiologic and immunologic perspective. *Journal of Athletic Training.* 1997;32(4):344-349.

7. Peters EM. Exercise, immunology and upper respiratory tract infections. *Int J Sports Med.* 1997;18:S69-S77.

8. Sevier TL. Infectious disease in athletes. *Med Clin North Am.* 1994;78(2):389-412.

9. Weidner TG. Upper respiratory illness and sport and exercise. *Int J Sports Med.* 1994;15(1):1-9.

10. Weidner TG, Sevier TL. Sport, exercise, and the common cold. *Journal of Athletic Training.* 1996;31(2):154-159.

11. Arnheim DD, Prentice WE. Other health conditions related to sports. In: Arnheim DD, Prentice WE, eds. *Principles of Athletic Training.* 8th ed. St. Louis, Mo: Mosby-Year Book; 1993:796-819.

12. O'Connor FG, Kugler JP, Oriscello RG. Sudden death in young athletes: screening for the needle in a haystack. *Am Fam Physician.* 1998;57(11):2763-2770.

13. Futterman LG, Myerburg R. Sudden death in athletes: an update. *Sports Med.* 1998;26(5):335-350.

14. Basilico FC. Cardiovascular disease in athletes. *Am J Sports Med.* 1999;27(1):108-121.

15. Garson AJ. Arrhythmias and sudden cardiac death in elite athletes. *Pediatria Medica E Chirurgica.* 1998;20:101-103.

16. Maron BJ, Isner JM, McKenna WJ. 26th Bethesda Conference: recommendations for determining eligibility for competition in athletes with cardiovascular abnormalities, task force 3: hypertrophic cardiomyopathy, myocarditis, and other myopericardial diseases and mitral valve prolapse. *Med Sci Sports Exerc.* 1994;26(10):S261-S267.

17. Nichols AW. Nonorthopedic problems in the aquatic athlete. *Clin Sports Med.* 1999;18(2):395-411.

18. Boyce TG. Gastroenteritis. In: Beers MH, Berkow R, eds. *The Merck Manual of Diagnosis and Therapy.* 17th ed. Whitehouse Station, NJ: Merck Research Laboratories; 1999:283-292.

19. Allen DB. Effects of fitness training on endocrine systems in children and adolescents. *Adv Pediatr.* 1999;46:41-66.

20. Johnson MB, Thiese SM. A review of overtraining syndrome: recognizing the signs and symptoms. *Journal of Athletic Training.* 1992;27(4):352-354.

21. Buxton BP, Daniell JE, Buxton BHJ, et al. Prevention of hepatitis B virus in athletic training. *Journal of Athletic Training.* 1994;29(2):107-112.

22. Bickley LS, Hoekelman RA. *Bates' Guide to Physical Examination and History Taking.* 7th ed. Philadelphia, Pa: Lippincott, Williams & Wilkins; 1999.

23. Fincher AL. Use of the otoscope in the evaluation of common injuries and illnesses of the ear. *Journal of Athletic Training.* 1994;29(1):52-59.

24. Arnheim DD, Prentice WE. Skin disorders. In: Arnheim DD, Prentice WE, eds. *Principles of Athletic Training.* 8th ed. St. Louis, Mo: Mosby-Year Book; 1993:420-452.

25. Fekety R, Sparling PK. Bacterial diseases. In: Beers MH, Berkow R, eds. *The Merck Manual of Diagnosis and Therapy.* 17th ed. Whitehouse Station, NJ: Merck Research Laboratories; 1999: 1147-1209.

26. Arnold BL. A review of selected blood-borne pathogen position statements and Federal regulations. *Journal of Athletic Training.* 1995;30(2):171-176.

27. Brkich M. Infectious waste disposal plan of the high school athletic trainer. *Journal of Athletic Training.* 1995;30(3):208-209.

28. National Athletic Trainers' Association Board of Directors. Blood-borne pathogens guidelines for athletic trainers. *Journal of Athletic Training.* 1995;30(3):203-204.

Chapter Eleven

Oncology

PURPOSES

- Describe the etiology and pathophysiological mechanisms of cancer.
- Discuss medical history findings relevant to cancer.
- Identify signs and symptoms of cancer, including early warning signs of potential cancer.
- Perform physical examination tasks relevant to cancer.
- Discuss, compare, and contrast common types of cancer.

INTRODUCTION

This chapter reviews the signs and symptoms of cancers that may be encountered among young (ages 5 to 50), physically active persons. This should provide athletic trainers with a basic awareness and understanding of cancer and its associated warning signs. Roles of athletic trainers with respect to persons with cancer involve early detection, education, and following precautions for physical activity. Knowledge of the etiology, mechanisms, and signs and symptoms of cancer of various organ systems facilitates early detection. Educating students and athletes to recognize warning signs and self-examination techniques may allow them to identify potential cancer and seek a medical examination. Finally, for persons recovering from cancer or who are in remission (recovery such that no active disease is detectable), athletic trainers should be aware of the relative precautions and contraindications relative to physical activity.

REVIEW OF PHYSIOLOGY AND PATHOGENESIS

Cancer, defined as pathological cell growth and proliferation, ultimately affects one in four people. One-third of all persons diagnosed with cancer survive at least 5 years after identification of the disease (5 years is the minimal time for estimating cancer survival rates).[1] Cancers form tumors in affected organs, although not all tumors are cancerous. Benign tumors are often only abnormal accumulations of normal cells (hyperplasia) and may not be harmful. Benign tumors grow slowly and act like the cells in the tissue of origin. Malignant tumors, however, consist of undifferentiated, or nonspecific, cells. These cells do not function like cells of the original tissue but instead divide very rapidly due to abnormal chromosomal composition (dysplasia).[2] Malignant tumors are progressive and invasive, interfering with the function of normal cells in the affected organ or system.

Cancer can occur in virtually any system of the body. As noted above, abnormal chromosomes cause proliferation. These chromosomal defects can be inherited or acquired through exposure to environmental carcinogens (substances known to cause genetic mutation). The abnormal cells do not function properly and replicate at a very high rate. Eventually, healthy, functional cells are either completely replaced by cancerous cells or the resulting tumor grows large enough to impair the organ or other surrounding structures (such as blood vessels or nerves). Cancer cells may also migrate to other tissues in adjacent or associated systems, a process called metastasis. Cancer metastases spread to multiple sites, most commonly the spine, lungs, and brain, subsequently causing tumors and impairment of function in those organs.[2] Once cancer has metastasized, prognosis (probable recovery or outcome) becomes significantly worse.

Certain risk factors increase the opportunity for cancer to develop, including a positive family history, smoking, high-fat low-fiber diet, chronic alcohol use, prolonged exposure to sunlight, psychoemotional stress, occupation, and gender (for certain cancers).[1] This chapter reviews signs and symptoms of cancers of various systems, with emphasis on those most common among physically active persons.

Table 11-1

AMERICAN CANCER SOCIETY'S WARNING SIGNS FOR POTENTIAL CANCER

- Change in bowel or bladder habits
- Unusual bleeding or discharge
- Indigestion or difficulty swallowing
- Persistent cough or hoarseness
- Nonhealing wound(s)
- Thickening of tissue (particularly breast)
- Change in wart or mole

SIGNS AND SYMPTOMS

As a result of inflammation, most cancers cause fever and pain. Cancer eventually interferes with organ function and thus can produce any of the signs and symptoms of specific systems discussed in Chapters Three through Eight. Table 11-1 gives warning signs of potential cancer, as outlined by the American Cancer Society.

Fever

Cancer can produce a low-grade fever in response to increased metabolic activity in cancer cells and the immune system.

Fatigue

Increased demand for energy and the catabolism of muscle and other tissues cause a persistent and progressive fatigue and decreased tolerance for activity.

Lymphadenopathy

Lymphomas are cancers that originate and proliferate in the lymph nodes and lymphatic system, producing swelling in multiple lymph nodes. In addition, the lymph nodes are common sites of metastasis for many types of cancer.

Night Symptoms

Pain, diaphoresis, or other symptoms that wake a person during the night may be an early sign of cancer. Organ systems dominated by parasympathetic control, such as gastrointestinal, hepatic-biliary, and renal-urogenital, are more active at night and may therefore become more symptomatic when affected by cancer.

Cyclical Pain Pattern

Intermittent pain cycles may regularly reflect pathology of organ systems that function in such a manner (eg, gastrointestinal, hepatic-biliary, and renal-urogenital). In addition, symptoms associated with certain body functions, such as digestion (following a meal), urination, or breathing, may be associated with underlying cancer in that system.

Unusual Muscle and Joint Pain

Muscle or joint pain that does not change with posture or movement and becomes progressively worse over time suggests serious underlying pathology, potentially including cancer.

Pain Patterns

An organ system that develops cancer may produce signs and symptoms related to that system. Secondary signs and symptoms, however, commonly arise in other systems, including the lungs, bone, brain, and CNS once metastasis has occurred. Sometimes signs and symptoms at the sites of metastases are noticed before those of the primary system. Pain patterns are identical to those outlined in Chapters Three through Eight.

Medical History and Physical Examination

Family and Personal History

Family history can be a significant risk factor for certain cancers, particularly those of the breast, ovary, and colon. Personal history may reveal presence of the warning signs and symptoms for cancer (see Table 11-1). The symptomatic course is important, including cycle (rhythm), intensity, and duration of symptoms, as well as how much time has passed since the symptoms originated.

Inspection

Changes in appearance or size of moles and mucous membranes can indicate cancerous changes. New, growing, or tender masses, lymphadenopathy, and nonhealing wounds occur with certain types of cancer. Tumors (neoplasms) of bone or connective tissue often become large enough to palpate. Tumors in the abdomen may also be palpable, although considerable practice and skill is necessary to discern normal anatomy from pathology (see Lab Activity Six).

Physical Examination

Signs of cancer are usually associated with the tissue, organ, or system of origin or tumor site. Many of the signs presented in Chapters Three through Eight may appear, depending on which system the cancer affects. Signs of general illness, including fever, malaise, and weight loss, are also often present.

PATHOLOGY AND PATHOGENESIS

Testicular Cancer

Testicular cancer is the most common cancer among males aged 15 to 35. Although primarily genetic in nature, a history of cryptorchidism (see Chapter Seven), significant testicular trauma or infection, and infertility are risk factors for the development of testicular cancer. Although usually detectable upon regular self-exam as progressive, unilateral testicular swelling, the disease may go unrecognized until metastases in the spine cause back pain or other symptoms such as abdominal pain, fatigue, weight loss, or nausea.[3] Early detection is critical for long-term survival. Metastases in the spine indicate poor prognosis.

Prostate Cancer

Prostate cancer is primarily a disease of aging males, becoming progressively more common each decade after age 50. Prostate cancer causes the third most cancer deaths among men (after lung and colon cancer), with metastases in the spine, pelvis, hips, lung, and liver very common and often the first indication of disease.[3] As tumor size increases, the urethra becomes progressively obstructed and urinary function becomes impaired. Back pain, dysuria, and nocturia in middle-aged men suggests prostate enlargement, which may be a result of prostate cancer or benign prostate changes with age (benign prostatic hypertrophy).[3] A history of diagnosed prostate cancer increases the probability of vertebral metastasis. If history is suspicious for prostate involvement, the person should be referred to his physician for x-rays and medical testing.

Cervical, Ovarian, and Uterine Cancers

Cancers of the female reproductive system occur primarily in women over age 45 and are typically asymptomatic until metastases exist. Unusual vaginal bleeding or discharge (nonmenstrual or postmenopausal) may be the only indication of underlying disease. Precancerous changes in the cervix can be detected during routine annual medical examination with a medical test called a Pap smear, which has lead to much higher survival rates.

Unfortunately, ovarian and uterine cancers have very low survival rates since they are difficult to detect until they are very advanced.[4,5] Risk factors for these cancers include a history of numerous sexual partners, postmenopausal estrogen supplementation, endocrine disorders, never becoming pregnant, family history, and an age of 40 years or older.[4-6]

Breast Cancer

Breast cancer is the second most common malignancy among women (lung cancer is first).[2] A positive family history increases risk and is associated with an earlier age of onset.[2,7] Hormonal factors are also involved since women who have never been pregnant or who have a first child after age 35, both of which affect female hormone levels, are at increased risk.[2,7] Breast cancer typically occurs in women over age 45, but appearance at an earlier age usually indicates greater severity of the disease.

The first physical sign of breast cancer is a palpable lump in the breast tissue.[4,7] In addition, the breast may be unusually tender, display dimpling (particularly around the nipple), or produce discharge from the nipple.[2,4] Common sites of metastasis from breast cancer include the bones of the ribs, vertebrae, or hips.[7] Regular self-examination should be conducted at least monthly, beginning in late adolescence. An estimated 90% of breast lesions are discovered in this manner. Regular mammography (radiographic imaging of the breast) should begin between ages 35 and 40 years and be repeated biannually until age 50, then repeated annually thereafter.[6] Mammography and other imaging tests may identify breast cancer before it becomes a palpable tumor.

Lung Cancer

Lung cancer causes more cancer-related deaths in the United States among both genders than any other type of cancer.[2,8] The rate of lung cancer varies proportionately with the rate of smoking in the population; a higher rate of smoking produces a higher rate of lung cancer. Up to 90% of lung cancer occurs in persons who smoke. Smoking is thus a major risk factor for development of lung cancer.[2,8,9] Smoking and use of other tobacco products also greatly increases the risk of oral and throat cancers.[1] Chronic exposure to other chemicals (asbestos, hydrocarbons, polyethylenes, etc) and radiation also greatly increases the risk of lung cancer.[8,9]

Lung cancer is rarely diagnosed before age 35, most frequently occurring among people over age 45. In early stages, pulmonary symptoms may be mild, such as a persistent productive cough, which is so common among people who smoke that it may be ignored.[9] As the lung cancer advances, loss of appetite, weight loss, and fatigue (from loss of pulmonary function) may occur.[8,9] Depending on the location of the tumor within the lung, dyspnea, stridor, pneumonia, pleurisy, and hemoptysis may appear.[2] A tumor in the superior lung may grow large enough to impinge on the brachial plexus, causing shoulder and arm pain.[8] Diagnosis is made with chest x-rays and laboratory tests.

Treatment is surgical resection of the affected portion of the lung, radiation therapy, chemotherapy, or a combination of these techniques. Treatment depends on the stage and extent of the tumor. Due to difficult early detection, prognosis is generally poor.[9] Less than 15% of patients survive 5 years after diagnosis. Bony metastases are very common and may cause chest (ribs), neck, or back (vertebrae) pain. The lungs also commonly develop metastatic tumors from cancer of other organs.[9]

Leukemia

Leukemia describes cancer of bone marrow cells and is characterized by production of undeveloped white blood cells (WBCs).[2,10] These abnormal WBCs do not respond to infection normally, so immune system function is compromised.[10,11] In addition, the high rate of proliferation of WBC in bone marrow inhibits formation of red blood cells (RBCs) and platelets, thus causing anemia and clotting disorders (see Chapter Three).[2,11] Leukemia can be acute, producing rapid deterioration, or chronic pain with a slower progression.

Major signs of all leukemias are anemia, chronic recurrent infections, and abnormal bleeding from the gums, nose, or in mid-menstrual cycle.[10] Additional signs and symptoms depend on other affected organs. Chronic leukemia can cause systemic signs (fatigue, weight loss, low-grade fever), dyspnea, and easy bruising. Acute leukemia produces profuse bleeding, lymphadenopathy, hepatomegaly, splenomegaly, deep bone pain, headache, high-grade fever, cranial nerve effects (see Chapter Eight), and vomiting.[2,10,11] Unless treated appropriately, all leukemias are fatal. Chemotherapy and bone marrow transplant are the main methods of treatment. Leukemia may go into remission for many years, then recur and cause death within weeks or months. Early diagnosis techniques and advances in treatment have been able to cure leukemia in many patients.

Hodgkin's Lymphoma

Hodgkin's lymphoma (Hodgkin's disease) is a relatively rare malignancy that develops in one or more lymph nodes during adolescence or early adulthood.[2,10] The disease metastasizes to many lymph nodes and organs, including the spleen, liver, lungs, and bone.[2,11] Most commonly, the first sign is painless, large lymph nodes, palpated as firm, movable masses in the unilateral groin or neck.[2] General systemic signs and symptoms may also be present. In untreated, advanced stages, chronic recurrent infections and multiple symptomatic metastases occur.[11] With early recognition, Hodgkin's disease is treated with radiation and chemotherapy and has a very good prognosis.[2] Non-Hodgkin's lymphoma, another form of lymphatic cancer, presents clinical signs and symptoms similar to Hodgkin's, but the disease is usually more widespread, aggressive, and has a worse prognosis. Hence, lymph node swelling, particularly if reported as persisting more than a couple of weeks, requires medical referral.

Colorectal Cancer

The third most common cancer (after lung and breast) and second most common cause of cancer-related death is colorectal cancer, with risk increasing with age.[2,12,13] Risk also increases for those with previous or existing colon disease, previous cancer of the breast or female urogenital system, and a positive family history.[2,12] A diet high in fat and sugar but low in fiber has also been associated with development of colorectal cancer.[12-14] Fifty to 75% of colorectal tumors occur in the sigmoid colon or rectum.[12,14]

Early symptoms include change in bowel habits (either diarrhea, constipation, or both) and intermittent cramping pain.[2,12,13,15] Hematochezia or frank blood in the stool may occur in later stages, causing an iron-deficiency anemia (see Chapter Three).[12] Increasing tumor size may also cause abdominal, back, or pelvis pain, at which stage they are usually palpable during abdominal examination.[2,14] Constipation, nausea, vomiting, and abdominal distention occur as the bowel becomes progressively obstructed.[2] Presence of these signs and symptoms obviously requires a physician's examination. Surgical removal of the affected colon and radiation or chemotherapy (particularly for common liver and bone metastases) are the usual treatment.[12-14] Early detection and treatment can lead to a 5-year survival rate over 70%. Late stage with metastases and lymph node involvement decreases survival to 30%.[14]

Brain Cancer

Brain cancer is relatively prevalent among all age groups and is the second most common cause of cancer death among children. In addition, the brain is one of the most common sites for cancer metastases from other organ systems. Brain tumors cause increased pressure and interruption of nerve pathways.[16,17] Increased intracranial pressure produces headache, severe vomiting (without nausea), altered cognition, syncope, seizure, blurred vision, or cranial nerve signs (see Chapter Eight). Some patients are essentially asymptomatic, however, until their disease is quite advanced. Cancerous disruption of nervous pathways may cause ataxia, paralysis, dysarthria, paresthesia, behavioral changes, or signs of upper-level neuron impairment (see Chapter Eight).[17] Generally, 5-year survival rates exceed 70% for primary brain cancer if detected and treated appropriately with surgery, radiation, or chemotherapy.[16,17] Metastatic brain (or spinal) tumors treated primarily by radiation generally produce substantial residual impairment and disability with a relatively poor prognosis.

Skeletal Cancers

Osteoid Osteoma/Osteoblastoma

These benign but painful bone tumors may impair joint motion or impinge nerves or blood vessels as they grow.[7] Most frequent under age 30, recurrent dull, aching pain that increases at night and nearly completely disappears with anti-inflammatory use suggests osteoid osteoma or osteoblastoma.[7] Treatment is surgical excision. After postoperative healing and rehabilitation, return to full unlimited activity can be anticipated.

Other benign tumors that occur in bone are osteochondroma and chondroblastoma, both of which are clinically similar to osteoid osteoma and osteoblastoma and are treated symptomatically and surgically (including bone grafting) as needed.[7] Generally recovery is complete, although lengthy if large sections of bone are involved.

Osteosarcoma and Chondrosarcoma

These malignant tumors occur in the metaphysis of long bones and articular cartilage, respectively.[2,7] Osteosarcoma is most common among adolescent and young adult males, whereas chondrosarcoma presents more often among middle-aged adults.[2] Osteosarcoma has an affinity for rapidly growing epiphyses, often in the distal femur, and causes pain, swelling, and joint impairment without a history of injury. Pathological fracture may also occur if the bone is sufficiently weakened.[2] Metastases to the lungs and brain occur early in osteosarcoma and are associated with a worse prognosis.[2]

In contrast, chondrosarcoma progresses more slowly and is less likely to metastasize. Clinical signs are few, with a gradually increasing tender bone mass as the most frequent sign. Prognosis is considerably better than that of osteosarcoma. Recent diagnosis and treatment advances continue to increase the survival rates for both tumors.[2,7]

Multiple Myeloma

Multiple myeloma is a bone marrow tumor that develops slowly, usually during middle to late adulthood. Bone pain in the back, pelvis, or ribs, either as an intermittent mild ache or as sudden excruciating pain, are usual first symptoms.[10] X-rays show characteristic "punched-out bone" lesions.[2,10] Pathological fractures and skeletal deformities may occur, producing neurological signs, symptoms, and impairment.[2,10] Systemic signs and signs of anemia occur if blood cell production is impaired by the diseased bone marrow.[10] Bone degeneration leads to metabolic imbalances, including hypercalcemia (high levels of calcium in the blood), hyperuricemia (high levels of uric acid in the blood), dehydration (from vomiting and frequent urination), and renal impairment (see Chapter Seven).[2,10] Treatment includes anti-inflammatories, analgesics, chemotherapy, and bone marrow transplantation. Notoriously difficult to treat, less than 10% of patients with multiple myeloma survive 10 years after diagnosis.[10]

Recovery and Remission

Return to activity during or after recovery from cancer depends on several factors, including extent and duration of the disease, patient age, type of cancer, presence of metastases and related complications, and overall health and fitness prior to onset of disease. With nearly all types of cancer, deconditioning occurs from relative inactivity during the illness and metabolic muscle wasting accompanies the severe illness and is a side effect of medical treatments (chemotherapy, radiation, and surgery). Although many people survive cancer and return to very active lives, the recovery process is extremely individual. The athletic trainer should consult the attending oncologist or primary care physician to obtain specific precautions or contraindications relative to the desired level of physical activity.

Pediatric Concerns

Acute Lymphoblastic Leukemia

Acute lymphoblastic leukemia (ALL) is the most common form of childhood leukemia. ALL appears most often in early childhood (under 5 years of age).[11] Signs and symptoms follow those outlined for acute leukemia above. Bone pain in the chest or tibia is also common. Clinical presentation of ALL is initially suggestive of acute infection, with high-grade fever and rapid physical collapse. ALL is a medical emergency, but timely treatment leads to a 75% 5-year survival rate.

Ewing's Sarcoma

Ewing's sarcoma can affect any part of the bone, usually appearing in the lower extremity. This is the most common malignancy in children, with most cases diagnosed before the age of 20 years. Nontraumatic pain of the affected region is the main symptom, accompanied by limb swelling and a low-grade fever.[18] A tender mass may be palpable over the bone in more advanced stages. Neurologic signs and symptoms occur if the tumor impinges a nerve.[2] Like other bone cancers, treatment consists of radiation, chemotherapy, and surgery, including widescale tissue resection or amputation as necessary to remove all cancerous cells. Between 50% and 70% of children with Ewing's sarcoma survive at least 5 years, with better prognosis for earlier diagnosis and lack of metastases.[2,18] Ewing's sarcoma is detectable by routine x-ray. Any child or adolescent with unexplained, vague limb or joint pain should be promptly referred for appropriate diagnostic testing.

Summary

Cancer is pathological proliferation of undifferentiated cells that forms malignant tumors. The tumors impair normal organ system function. Cancer produces signs and symptoms of both general illness and specific to a particular system, presenting a clinical "picture" of chronic or acute severe illness. Athletic trainers should be aware of risk factors and early warning signs for cancer. In addition, they should be aware of potential precautions for physical activity for persons recovering from cancer. Education of students, athletes, and patients with respect to warning signs and self-examination techniques may help them detect cancer in earlier stages, thereby increasing probability and duration of survival.

RESOURCES

Cancer

- American Cancer Society. www.cancer.org
- atlife.com cancer site. atcancer.com/cancer
- Mammacare.com site containing a "scientifically validated" system on how to instruct women to conduct self-examination of the breast. www.mammacare.com
- Yahoo directory. dir.yahoo.com/Health/Diseases_and_Conditions/Cancers

REFERENCES

1. Goodman CC. Oncology. In: Goodman CC, Boissonnault WG, eds. *Pathology: Implications for the Physical Therapist*. Philadelphia, Pa: WB Saunders Company; 1998:152-172.

2. Goodman CC, Snyder TEK. Overview of oncologic signs and symptoms. In: Goodman CC, Snyder TEK, eds. *Differential Diagnosis in Physical Therapy: Musculoskeletal and Systemic Conditions*. 3rd ed. Philadelphia, Pa: WB Saunders Company; 2000:334-389.

3. McLinn DM, Boissonnault WG. Screening for male urogenital system disease. In: Boissonnault WG, ed. *Examination in Physical Therapy Practice: Screening for Medical Disease*. 2nd ed. New York: Churchill Livingstone Inc; 1995:117-132.

4. Gould BE. Reproductive system disorders. *Pathophysiology for the Health-Related Professions*. Philadelphia, Pa: WB Saunders Company; 1997:428-452.

5. Gould BE. Neoplasms. *Pathophysiology for the Health-Related Professions*. Philadelphia, Pa: WB Saunders Company; 1997:54-69.

6. Boissonnault WG. The female genital/reproductive system. In: Goodman CC, Boissonnault WG, eds. *Pathology: Implications for the Physical Therapist*. Philadelphia, Pa: WB Saunders Company; 1998:559-568.

7. Randall T, McMahon K. Screening for musculoskeletal system disease. In: Boissonnault WG, ed. *Examination in Physical Therapy Practice: Screening for Medical Disease*. 2nd ed. New York: Churchill-Livingstone Inc.;1995:223-255.

8. Goodman CC. The respiratory system. In: Goodman CC, Boissonnault WG, eds. *Pathology: Implications for the Physical Therapist*. Philadelphia, Pa: WB Saunders Company; 1998:399-455.

9. Gould BE. Respiratory disorders. *Pathophysiology for the Health-Related Professions*. Philadelphia, Pa: WB Saunders Company; 1997:213-252.

10. Goodman CC. The hematologic system. In: Goodman CC, Boissonnault WG, eds. *Pathology: Implications for the Physical Therapist*. Philadelphia, Pa: WB Saunders Company; 1998:354-398.

11. Gould BE. Cardiovascular and lymphatic disorders. *Pathophysiology for the Health-Related Professions*. Philadelphia, Pa: WB Saunders Company; 1997:159-212.

12. Bass NM, Smith JHJ, Van Dyke RW. Neoplasms of the gastrointestinal tract. In: Andreoli TE, Carpenter CCJ, Plum F, et al, eds. *Cecil Essentials of Medicine*. 2nd ed. Philadelphia, Pa: WB Saunders Company; 1990:297-303.

13. Gould BE. Digestive system disorders. *Pathophysiology for the Health-Related Professions*. Philadelphia, Pa: WB Saunders Company; 1997:253-298.

14. Livstone EM. Tumors of the gastrointestinal tract: large-bowel tumors. In: Beers MH, Berkow R, eds. *The Merck Manual of Diagnosis and Therapy*. 17th ed. Whitehouse Station, NJ: Merck Research Laboratories; 1999:326-330.

15. DeGowin RL, Brown DD. *DeGowin's Diagnostic Examination*. 7th ed. New York: McGraw-Hill; 2000.

16. Gould BE. Neurologic disorders. *Pathophysiology for the Health-Related Professions*. Philadelphia, Pa: WB Saunders Company; 1997:320-376.

17. Konecne SM. Central nervous system neoplasms. In: Goodman CC, Boissonnault WG, eds. *Pathology: Implications for the Physical Therapist*. Philadelphia, Pa: WB Saunders Company; 1998:702-722.

18. Randall T. Musculoskeletal neoplasms. In: Goodman CC, Boissonnault WG, eds. *Pathology: Implications for the Physical Therapist*. Philadelphia, Pa: WB Saunders Company; 1998:639-659.

Chapter Twelve

Differentiation of Signs and Symptoms

PURPOSES

- Identify signs and symptoms of medical emergencies.
- Discuss signs and symptoms similar to musculoskeletal pathology found with systemic pathology.
- Review the process of differentiation.
- Present evaluation and management algorithms according to primary symptom.

INTRODUCTION

This chapter summarizes the preceding chapters' information into a clinical assessment scheme. Understanding pathophysiological mechanisms and clinical presentations of various diseases is important. It is equally important, however, to differentiate a medical emergency from less severe illnesses, as well as to distinguish musculoskeletal injury from systemic illness or disease. This chapter reviews which conditions or situations constitute a medical emergency that supersede the need to differentiate the system of origin. It next provides a method to evaluate illness or injury by the relative seriousness of the condition. Third, several tables list conditions of the various organ systems that may produce signs and symptoms similar to musculoskeletal conditions. Finally, algorithms organized by primary sign or symptom are presented as guides to assessment and clinical decision-making. If a topic is not fully understood, rereading the related chapters or sections is recommended. In addition, several medical references that were consulted frequently during development of this chapter can provide additional information.[1-9]

MEDICAL EMERGENCY

The conditions listed in Table 12-1 constitute a medical emergency, thus requiring rapid activation of emergency medical services (EMS) and transport to a medical facility. These conditions do not require a full differential assessment since the course of action would not change. Delay of appropriate treatment, however, may cause permanent tissue damage or death. The role of the athletic trainer in these situations, after recognition of the emergency, is to provide life support or basic first aid until EMS arrives or arrange transportation to a medical facility. Monitoring vital signs, treating for shock, splinting suspected fractures, and controlling severe bleeding are appropriate actions after EMS is activated. Noting the time of the incident and any known mechanism of injury may also be useful to medical personnel. Emergency plans should be established before the season or school year and reviewed regularly by sports medicine and coaching personnel.

EVALUATING THE SERIOUSNESS OF THE CONDITION

This section presents a framework for assessment to determine the relative severity of a condition, thus facilitating clinical decision-making (ie, referral to emergency, urgent, or standard/routine medical care). The section is organized from the most to the least severe situation and assumes the medical emergencies in Table 12-1 have been excluded during the primary assessment. Table 12-2 summarizes the assessment process when determining the seriousness of the condition.

The first and most serious pathological signs are abnormalities of the major life-sustaining functions, such as breathing and circulation. Heart rate, respiration rate, blood pressure, or body temperature (vital signs) outside the normal ranges, either high or low (Table 12-3), require prompt medical referral. Baseline values should be obtained during preparticipation examination of athletes. Significant changes from these baseline values demand medical explanation. Noticeable changes (ie, steady increase or decrease) over several minutes or hours may indicate rapidly progressing pathology. Many pathological conditions eventually

Table 12-1

MEDICAL EMERGENCIES: IMMEDIATELY ACTIVATE EMS

Condition	Signs and Symptoms	Management (After Activating EMS)
Rapid changes (within minutes) in vital signs	Significant changes in BP, HR, RR, body temperature	ABCs, monitor vital signs until EMS arrives
Shock	Systolic BP < 90 mmHg, tachycardia and hyperpnea, pallor, diaphoresis, cyanosis, altered cognition, lethargy	Elevate feet, ABCs, monitor vital signs
Nontraumatic syncope or unconsciousness	Complete loss of consciousness lasting over 1 minute	ABCs, monitor vital signs, mental and neurological tests if awakened (urgent referral if reported by subject but not observed by examiner)
Profuse bleeding or bleeding from mucous membranes or orifices	Large volume of bleeding that persists longer than 1 or 2 minutes	Treat for shock, apply pressure if possible
Abdominal rigidity or severe pain	Tenderness to palpation, unusual distention, palpable organs/mass	Assess for other systemic signs; monitor vital signs
Prolonged or unexplained severe vomiting or diarrhea	Accompanied by syncope, hematemesis, and fever	Prevent dehydration, treat for shock, monitor vital signs
Known or suspected poisoning	History of exposure, severe vomiting, headache, dyspnea, hypotension, altered consciousness, syncope, loss of motor coordination or control	Call poison control or read packaging if available
Seizure	No known history of epilepsy or previous seizure	Protect head, ABCs, remove to quiet area after seizure

ABCs = monitor airway, breathing, and circulation; EMS = emergency medical service; BP = blood pressure; HR = heart rate; RR = respiratory rate.

Table 12-2

HIERARCHY OF ASSESSMENT FOR SERIOUSNESS OF CONDITION

1. Vital signs	Changes in heart rate, respiration rate, blood pressure, body temperature
2. Brainstem and neuromotor	Smell, vision, hearing, taste, swallowing, speech, tactile sensation, reflexes, coordination, balance
3. Endocrine and metabolic	Dehydration, lethargy, fatigue, altered cognition, edema, loss or gain in body weight
4. Daily functions	Sleep, eating, urination, defecation, sexual function

Table 12-3

ABNORMALLY HIGH AND LOW VALUES FOR VITAL SIGNS

Vital Sign	High	Normal	Low
Heart rate (at rest)	> 100 bpm	70 to 100 bpm	< 60 bpm
Respiration rate (at rest)	> 20 bpm	10 to 15 bpm	< 10 bpm
Blood pressure	> 140 systolic > 90 diastolic	100 to 140 systolic 70 to 90 diastolic	< 90 systolic < 70 diastolic
Body temperature	< 96°F	97° to 99°F	< 100°F

bpm = beats per minute.

affect these vital body functions, making them useful indicators of potentially serious pathology.

Next, evaluation of brainstem (smell, vision, facial sensation and movement, hearing, taste, speech, and swallowing) and other neurological function (reflexes, coordination, ataxia, balance, sensation) is conducted. The brain and nervous system, like the heart and lungs, are very sensitive to changes in the internal environment of the body. Thus, impairment of neurological status usually indicates a significant pathological process. Furthermore, the neurological system allows perception and interaction with the environment. If these functions are impaired, the person may be unable to walk, drive, or perform other tasks safely. Rapid changes (minutes to hours) in neurological function suggests an urgent medical condition.

At the next level of severity, signs of endocrine or metabolic disorders are often subtle and therefore require careful examination. Fortunately, most endocrine-metabolic conditions develop more slowly than cardiopulmonary or neurological disorders. Potential indicators include gradual changes in body temperature, signs of dehydration (dry tongue, decreased skin turgor, tachycardia, postural hypotension), lethargy or fatigue, altered cognition, peripheral neuropathies (sensory or motor, usually bilaterally distributed), presence of edema, or a significant (more than 5% change) loss or gain in body weight. Certain metabolic conditions constitute a medical emergency, such as diabetic ketoacidosis (see Chapter Seven), but most develop slowly over several days. If untreated, however, the long-term consequences can be debilitating and permanent.

Changes in regulation or pattern of "normal" day-to-day functions, such as sleep (insomnia, hypersomnia, or sleep disrupted by symptoms), eating (loss of appetite or sudden polyphagia), urination or defecation (frequency and volume), and sexual function are yet more subtle and difficult to detect. A pathological condition, if serious enough, affects daily life. These effects may be the earliest indicators of a slowly developing chronic disease (eg, cancer, degenerative neurological disorders) but are difficult to observe due to their insidious and personal nature. Taking a careful medical history is required to assess this information accurately. Any change in the activities that the person mentions is significant, particularly if accompanied by other systemic signs and symptoms.

Tables 12-4 through 12-8 list pathological conditions by organ system that present signs or symptoms similar to musculoskeletal conditions. Table 12-9 lists psychological red flags that require urgent medical evaluation. Table 12-10 provides possible pathology by body region of symptoms, which could lead to confusion when differentiating musculoskeletal from systemic conditions.

ASSESSMENT ALGORITHMS FOR KEY SYMPTOMS

The following algorithms (set of rules for decision-making in table form) should be used to assist the clinical decision-making process. They are not intended to replace a physician's medical examination and diagnosis. If a person's signs and symptoms are suggestive of systemic pathology listed in the algorithms, the index of suspicion is raised enough to warrant medical referral. This does not mean the condition exists, only that it cannot be excluded without medical examination and testing. If in doubt, refer immediately. Record all pertinent findings in your referral report. Document your recommendation for referral in your medical record and when and to whom (eg, the athlete, parents, spouse, etc) instructions were provided. The presence of conditions and signs and symptoms in Table 12-1 always take precedence and should be excluded by primary assessment before performing additional evaluation. Any person who exhibits syncope, rapidly changing vital signs, or appears to be in shock should be transported by EMS immediately.

The algorithms outline a clinical assessment process for nonorthopedic pathology, but they do not substitute for sound judgment and experience. The usual secondary assessment procedure of medical history, inspection, palpation, and special testing should be followed but adjusted appropriately for the apparent nature and urgency of the condition. The information collected during the secondary assessment allows application of the algorithms and potentially better clinical decisions.

Algorithms work like flow charts. First, locate the algorithm titled with the key symptom of the patient's complaint (eg, Abdominal Pain). Beginning in the uppermost left corner, a list of accompanying signs or symptoms flows down the left side of the table, approximately in decreasing order of severity. If the secondary signs and symptoms are not present, follow the "No" down to the next sign or symptom. When one of these signs or symptoms matches the patient's condition, following the word "Yes" (ie, moving to the right on the table) provides

Table 12-4

CARDIOVASCULAR AND PULMONARY DISORDERS

Condition	Confounding Symptom	Differentiating Signs and Symptoms
Cardiac ischemia or valve stenosis	Left arm pain	Chest pain that worsens with activity; dyspnea, diaphoresis, or syncope; over age 35
Sickle-cell anemia	Leg pain	Abdominal pain, enlarged abdominal organs, nosebleeds, fever, headache; African-American male
Thoracic outlet syndrome or vascular occlusive disorder	Arm (or leg) pain	Pain worsens during activity and is relieved by rest; edema, paresthesia, fatigue in limb with exercise, distal cyanosis
Aortic aneurysm	Sudden severe or intermittent moderate back pain	Pain with mild activity or at rest; palpable, pulsating mass in abdomen; auscultated bruit in abdomen; nausea, cough, or paresthesia
Pneumothorax	Back or trunk pain	History of chest trauma, chest pain, severe dyspnea, tachypnea, hyperresonance upon percussion of thorax, absent breath sounds
Spleen injury	Left shoulder pain (Kehr's sign)	Painful or rigid LUQ to palpation, nausea, history of left thorax or abdominal trauma

LUQ = left upper abdominal quadrant

Table 12-5

GASTROINTESTINAL AND HEPATIC DISORDERS

Condition	Confounding Symptom	Differentiating Signs and Symptoms
Peptic ulcer	Thoracic, chest, or neck pain	Pain changes after eating, worse at night, loss of appetite or vomiting may occur; history of NSAID use, alcohol abuse, tobacco use, or psychological stress
Appendicitis	Back or right hip pain	Progressive worsening of condition, nausea, may be fever or fatigue, rebound tenderness of RLQ

Table 12-5 continued

Condition	Confounding Symptom	Differentiating Signs and Symptoms
Hernia	Anterior hip or thigh pain	Pain worse with activity, Valsalva's maneuver, or certain postures; tenderness or palpable mass at inguinal or femoral canal
Liver injury	Right shoulder pain	Painful or rigid RUQ to palpation, nausea, vomiting, history of right trauma to thorax or abdomen
Gallstones (cholelithiasis)	Right shoulder pain	Painful or rigid RUQ to palpation, nausea, vomiting, history of intolerance to fatty foods

NSAID = nonsteroidal anti-inflammatory drug; RLQ = right lower abdominal quadrant; RUQ = right upper abdominal quadrant.

Table 12-6

RENAL, UROGENITAL, AND ENDOCRINE DISORDERS

Condition	Confounding Symptom	Differentiating Signs and Symptoms
Kidney injury	Back or flank pain	History of trauma to abdomen or back, hematuria, painful percussion at costovertebral angle, edema of flank
Kidney stone (urolithiasis)	Back or groin pain	Nausea and vomiting, pallor, tachycardia, stable vital signs, positive family history
Prostatitis	Back pain	Pain unchanged by posture; nocturia, increased urgency and frequency of urination, difficulty initiating urine stream, male over age 50
Endometriosis	Back pain	Painful and heavy menstruation, painful sexual intercourse, female over age 30
Pregnancy	Back (or joint) pain	Amenorrhea, abdominal pain, recurrent nausea, weight gain, distal extremity edema, female beyond menarche; shock if ruptured ectopic pregnancy
Endocrine disorders	Widespread myalgia and arthralgia (depending on gland and affected hormone)	Weakness and atrophy, spasms, tachycardia/bradycardia, fatigue, paresthesias, dry or diaphoretic skin, slow healing

Table 12-7

NEUROLOGICAL AND PSYCHOLOGICAL DISORDERS

Condition	Confounding Symptom	Differentiating Signs and Symptoms
Spina bifida occulta	Back pain	Patch of hair over spine, absent spinous process upon palpation, normal neurological tests
Multiple sclerosis	Weakness or incoordination	Intermittent sensory and reflex changes, visual disturbance, unusual fatigue (particularly in heat), over age 20
Reflex sympathetic dystrophy	Severe localized pain	History of injury with joint immobilization, edema, decreased range of motion, skin and nail changes, increased skin temperature
Amyotropic lateral sclerosis	Weakness	Bilaterally symmetric weakness, hyperactive reflexes, over age 30
Guillain-Barré syndrome	Leg and back weakness and pain	Rapid progression (hours) headache, fever, history of recent viral infection, loss of reflexes
Myasthenia gravis	Sudden severe muscle fatigue	Rapid progression (hours), diplopia, dysarthria, dysphagia, dyspnea, normal reflexes; over age 20
Muscular dystrophy	Hip and shoulder weakness	Slowly progressive (years), frequent falls, difficulty rising from ground or with stairs, waddling gait age 8 to 12 years at onset
Child abuse	Multiple skin wounds, frequent unexplained injury, or multiple injuries in various stages of healing	Inconsistent or unreasonable history of injury, behavioral problems, difficulty interacting with peers, avoidance behaviors by child and family, substance abuse in family

a list of potential condition(s), with additional "confirmatory" signs and symptoms for the particular condition enclosed in parentheses. The recommended action for that condition is immediately to the right. The three actions are "ER" for emergency, indicating activation of EMS or other emergency plan, "Urgent" for conditions that are not emergencies but require medical attention in the next 24 to 36 hours, and "Standard" for conditions that require medical examination at the earliest convenience (eg, the next visit of the team physician), within a week.

Table 12-8

INFECTIONS, IMMUNE DISORDERS, AND CANCER

Condition	Confounding Symptom	Differentiating Signs and Symptoms
Meningitis	Severe neck pain	Headache, fever, neck rigidity, history of recent upper respiratory infection, vomiting, skin rash on head, altered mental status, rapid progression (hours)
Septic arthrosis and osteomyelitis	Joint or localized bone pain	Signs of acute inflammation, history of recent injury or surgery in the body region, fever (osteomyelitis), rapid progression (septic arthrosis)
Rheumatoid arthritis/juvenile RA	Bilateral hand or foot pain	Mild inflammation of affected joints, morning stiffness; adolescent age (jRA)
Urogenital cancers	Back or hip pain	Mild systemic signs, abdominal pain, abnormal urinary or sexual function (or menstruation in females); palpable mass (testicular or breast); testicular: male 15 to 35; prostate: male over 50; cervical, ovarian, uterine: female over 45; breast: female over 45
Lung cancer	Shoulder, arm, or neck pain	History of smoking, dyspnea, hemoptysis, pneumonia, over age 35
Leukemia or lymphoma	Deep "bone" pain	Frequent bleeding episodes, systemic signs, recurrent infection, anemia, lymphadenopathy, vomiting; most over age 10
Bone cancers	Dull, aching bone pain or tender bone mass	Impaired or painful joint function, signs of local inflammation or systemic signs

Some of the algorithms have the left column divided into subsections that specify a region of the body, an event, gender, or pattern of symptoms that assist in differentiating conditions. For instance, pregnancy is listed only under female. These left column subheadings are <u>underlined</u> for easier reference.

The word "AND" in all capital letters indicates that the signs or symptoms preceding and following both have to be present before proceeding to the "Yes" pathway. If both are not present, continue down the left column (following the "No"). The word "OR" in all capital letters indicates that at least one of the list of signs or symptoms separated by "OR's" must be present to proceed to the "Yes" pathway. All signs or symptoms preceding or following "OR" do not have to be present.

Table 12-9

PSYCHOLOGICAL RED FLAGS

- Disorientation
- Debilitating apathy or lethargy
- Sudden cognitive deficit
- Acquired memory deficit
- Permanent or rapidly alternating changes in affect (mood)
- Behavior dangerous to themselves or others
- Hallucination
- Severe agitation
- Violent behavior
- Confusion
- Antisocial or avoidance behavior

Table 12-10

POSSIBLE SYSTEMIC PATHOLOGY OF SYMPTOMS

Location of Symptoms	Possible Systemic Pathology
Left arm	Cardiac ischemia, spleen injury, lung cancer
Right arm	Liver injury, gallbladder disorder, lung cancer
Leg or groin pain	Sickle-cell anemia, appendicitis (right hip), hernia
Back or thoracic pain	Aortic aneurysm, pneumothorax, peptic ulcer, appendicitis, kidney disorder, prostatitis, endometriosis, pregnancy, spina bifida occulta, urogenital cancer
Neck pain	Meningitis, lung cancer
Multiple joints or sites	Endocrine disorder, child (or domestic) abuse, rheumatoid arthritis
Weakness or fatigue	Multiple sclerosis, amyotropic lateral sclerosis, Guillain-Barré syndrome, myasthenia gravis, muscular dystrophy

Bold words in the algorithms indicate that a separate algorithm exists for that specific sign or symptom. If a clinical decision is not reached by consulting one algorithm, another algorithm that coincides with another of the patient's complaints can be used.

REFERENCES

1. Andreoli TE, Carpenter CCJ, Plum F, et al, eds. *Cecil's Essentials of Medicine.* 2nd ed. Philadelphia, Pa: WB Saunders Company; 1990.

2. Beers MH, Berkow R, eds. *The Merck Manual of Diagnosis and Therapy.* 17th ed. Whitehouse Station, NJ: Merck Research Laboratories; 1999.

3. Bickley LS, Hoekelman RA. *Bates' Guide to Physical Examination and History Taking.* 7th ed. Philadelphia, Pa: Lippincott, Williams & Wilkins; 1999.

4. Daly S, Holmes PA, Blake GJ, et al, eds. *Professional Guide to Signs and Symptoms.* Springhouse, Pa: Springhouse Corporation; 1993.

5. DeGowin RL, Brown DD. *DeGowin's Diagnostic Examination.* 7th ed. New York: McGraw-Hill; 2000.

6. Gould BE. *Pathophysiology for the Health-Related Professions.* Philadelphia, Pa: WB Saunders Company; 1997.

7. Jamison JR. *Differential Diagnosis for Primary Practice.* London: Churchill Livingstone; 1999.

8. Shaw M, Roy CM, Bartelmo JM, et al, eds. *Pathophysiology Made Incredibly Easy.* Springhouse, Pa: Springhouse Corporation; 1998.

9. Underwood JCE, ed. *General and Systematic Pathology.* 2nd ed. New York: Churchill Livingstone; 1996.

ABDOMINAL PAIN

Accompanying Signs or Symptoms		Potential Condition (and Confirmatory S&S)	Action
Fever	Yes	See separate algorithm.	
No			
Vomiting or diarrhea?	Yes	See separate algorithm.	
No			
Rigidity OR rebound tenderness OR positive "jar" test OR signs of shock	Yes	Peritonitis, abdominal hemorrhage (eg, perforated ulcer, ruptured appendix)	ER
No			
Progressively worse AND distention OR rigidity OR worse when rising from supine	Yes	Peritonitis, abdominal hemorrhage (eg, perforated ulcer, ruptured appendix)	ER
No			
Absence of bowel sounds (>3 min)	Yes	Bowel obstruction (visible peristalsis, "tinkling" in proximal bowel, silence in distal bowel, status rapidly deteriorates)	ER

If none of the above, assess by the location of symptoms in the abdomen.

ABDOMINAL PAIN CONTINUED

Accompanying Signs or Symptoms		Potential Condition (and Confirmatory S&S)	Action
Epigastric or general abdominal			
Severe pain and hx Marfan's syndrome?	Yes	Aortic aneurysm (pulsing pain, does not decrease, cardiac signs)	ER
No			
Decreasing blood pressure, syncope, **chest pain**, or **dyspnea**?	Yes	Cardiovascular event (tachycardia, hyperpnea)	ER
No			
Chronic, recurs after meals?	Yes	Peptic ulcer	Standard
No			
Chronic, gnawing, night pain, vague location?	Yes	Pancreatitis or pancreatic tumor	Urgent
No			
Burning, worse with caffeine, spices, alcohol, when supine?	Yes	Esophageal reflux, peptic ulcer	Standard
No			
Distention, borborygmi, usually after ingestion of dairy products	Yes	Lactose intolerance	Standard
Suprapubic female (postmenarche)			
Amenorrhea and unusual vaginal discharge?	Yes	Miscarriage (known pregnancy) or ruptured ectopic pregnancy OR ruptured ovarian/uterine cysts (both progress to shock)	ER ER
No			
Amenorrhea, nausea, recent weight gain?	Yes	Pregnancy	Standard
No			
Unusual vaginal discharge?	Yes	Ovarian/uterine cysts, STD, UTI	Urgent
No			
Currently menstruating, referred to back/thighs, no fever?	Yes	Menstrual cramps (young or nonparous females)	Standard
No			
Recurrent, worse with menstruation?	Yes	Endometriosis (if unusual vaginal discharge, urgent)	Standard
Either gender			
Dysuria or **Hematuria**?	Yes	See separate algorithm.	

ABDOMINAL PAIN CONTINUED

Accompanying Signs or Symptoms		Potential Condition (and Confirmatory S&S)	Action
No			
With groin pain and **vomiting**?	Yes	Strangulated hernia	ER
No			
With flank or groin pain, incapacitating in intensity, and recurring at regular intervals?	Yes	Kidney stone (usually **hematuria** or **vomiting**)	ER
Right upper quadrant			
Trauma to right side/flank AND palpable rib fracture OR positive compression test	Yes	Possible liver, kidney damage	ER
No			
AND tender, rigid RUQ, without hematuria	Yes	Ruptured liver (falling BP, shock, right shoulder pain)	ER
No			
AND tender, rigid RUQ, with hematuria	Yes	Ruptured or contused right kidney	ER
No			
No history of trauma			
Severe cramping and rigidity with intermittent full relief?	Yes	Cholelithiasis (right shoulder pain, pain worse with deep breath, pain with percussion RUQ)	ER
No			
Diffuse, vague pain, tender RUQ AND positive hammering RUQ?	Yes	Cholecystitis, hepatitis (right shoulder or scapula pain)	Urgent
No			

Recheck for fever, vomiting, diarrhea, rebound tenderness, rigidity, distention, and bowel sounds (see top of chart); if still negative, see "epigastric or general abdominal" and "suprapubic" above.

Left upper quadrant			
Trauma to left side/flank AND palpable rib fracture OR positive compression test	Yes	Possible spleen, kidney damage	ER
No			
AND tender, rigid LUQ, without hematuria?	Yes	Ruptured spleen	ER
No			

Abdominal Pain continued

Accompanying Signs or Symptoms		Potential Condition (and Confirmatory S&S)	Action
AND tender, rigid LUQ, with hematuria?	Yes	Ruptured or contused left kidney	ER
No			

Recheck for fever, vomiting, diarrhea, rebound tenderness, rigidity, distention, and bowel sounds (see top of chart); if still negative, see "epigastric or general abdominal" and "suprapubic" above.

<u>Right lower quadrant</u>

Vomiting, pain originated in epigastric region?	Yes	Appendicitis in "intermediate" stage (tender McBurney's sign, positive rebound) OR inflammatory bowel disease OR ("Meckel's") diverticulitis (ER since these conditions cannot be differentiated through clinical examination alone)	ER ER
No			
Vomiting, positive rebound, positive "jar," rigidity	Yes	Perforated appendix (shock, fever) OR perforated ulcer (drains to RLQ)	ER
No			

Recheck for fever, vomiting, diarrhea, rebound tenderness, rigidity, distention, and bowel sounds (see top of chart); if still negative, see "epigastric or general abdominal" and "suprapubic" above.

<u>Left lower quadrant</u>

Tender LLQ, no rigidity	Yes	Diverticulitis or inflammatory bowel disease (usually hx of difficult defecation, alternating constipation and diarrhea)	Urgent
		if a fever is also present	ER
No			
Nontender mass in LLQ And reports straining to defecate small stools	Yes	Constipation	Standard
No			

Recheck for fever, vomiting, diarrhea, rebound tenderness, rigidity, distention, and bowel sounds (see top of chart); if still negative, see "epigastric or general abdominal" and "suprapubic" above.

BONE OR JOINT PAIN (NONTRAUMATIC)

Accompanying Signs or Symptoms		*Potential Condition* (and Confirmatory S&S)	*Action*
Fever	Yes	See separate algorithm.	
No			
Skin rash, **lymphadenitis**, fatigue, night pain, OR any other systemic signs?	Yes	Metabolic bone disease or tumor	Urgent
No			
Multiple joints involved AND significant morning stiffness?	Yes	Rheumatoid arthritis, Juvenile RA (age < 20 years)	Standard
No			
Recent injury OR orthopedic surgery in region			
AND mild inflammation?	Yes	Osteomyelitis (usually **fever**)	Urgent
AND severe inflammation, rapid onset?	Yes	Septic arthrosis (may not be a **fever**)	ER/Urgent
No			
Excruciating, severe inflammation, rapid onset, but no trauma?	Yes	Gout (progressively worsens)	Urgent
No			
Signs of neurological or vascular impairment (paresthesia, pallor, pulses or reflexes, OR specific motor weakness)			
AND rapid onset after injury or prolonged exercise?	Yes	Acute compartment syndrome	ER
AND recurrent with exercise, completely resolves with rest?	Yes	Chronic compartment syndrome	Standard
AND constant pain, slowly progressing in intensity?	Yes	Impingement or entrapment	Standard
No			
Night pain, nearly complete relief with NSAIDs, age < 30?	Yes	Osteoid osteoma, osteoblastoma	Urgent
No			
Tender mass palpable on bone			
AND inflamed, impaired joint, age < 30?	Yes	Osteosarcoma	Urgent
No			

BONE OR JOINT PAIN (NONTRAUMATIC) CONTINUED

Accompanying Signs or Symptoms		Potential Condition (and Confirmatory S&S)	Action
AND inflamed, impaired joint, age > 30?	Yes	Chondrosarcoma	Urgent
No			
AND inflamed, impaired joint, fever, age < 20?	Yes	Ewing's sarcoma	Urgent
No			
AND in spine, ribs, pelvis, systemic signs, and age > 30?	Yes	Multiple myeloma	Urgent
No			

Perform assessment for musculoskeletal condition or other systemic involvement (by location of symptoms) and refer appropriately.

CHEST PAIN

Accompanying Signs or Symptoms		Potential Condition (and Confirmatory S&S)	Action
Fever?	Yes	See separate algorithm.	
No			
Pain ≥ 15 min AND age ≥ 35 years? OR no improvement with rest? OR history of heart disease, diabetes, Marfan's?	Yes	Myocardial infarction or cardiac event (diaphoresis, left arm pain, **nausea**, denial, syncope, or anxiety)	ER
No			
Dyspnea, hemoptysis, cyanosis with sudden onset?	Yes	Pneumothorax (auscultation, percussion abnormal, tracheal deviation) or pulmonary embolism (hx suggests DVT; falling BP)	ER
No			
Syncope (hx or observed)? OR Unequal femoral or brachial pulses?	Yes	Cardiac event or aortic dissection	ER
No			
Tachycardia, hyperpnea, gasping breaths?	Yes	Tracheal or bronchial spasm (recent toxic exposure, hx asthma)	ER
AND pruritis (itching)?	Yes	Anaphylaxis (allergic reaction)	ER
No			
Recent or current infection (GI, URI, etc)	Yes	Pericarditis, endocarditis, pleurisy (fever, auscultated friction rub, systemic signs)	ER
No			

CHEST PAIN CONTINUED

Accompanying Signs or Symptoms		Potential Condition (and Confirmatory S&S)	Action
Dyspnea only with exertion?	Yes	Ischemic heart failure	Urgent
No			
Palpitations with exertion?	Yes	Arrythmia	Urgent
No			
Purulent **cough** AND abnormal auscultation?	Yes	Pneumonia or pulmonary infection (usually accompanied by fever)	Urgent
No			
Dysphagia that changes with meals, while reclining?	Yes	Upper GI; dyspepsia, gastric reflux (intermittent, recurrent, pain referring to left chest or arm)	Standard
No			
Palpable mass in chest muscle/skin?	Yes	Breast tumor or other neoplasm	Standard
No			
Single dermatome distribution?	Yes	Nerve root irritation	Standard
No			
Tender palpation of ribs, pectoralis, or costal cartilage?	Yes	Musculoskeletal injury (hx trauma, heavy lifting, previous episode)	Standard

COUGH

Accompanying Signs or Symptoms		Potential Condition (and Confirmatory S&S)	Action
Fever	Yes	See separate algorithm	
No			
Cyanosis	Yes	Airway obstruction, respiratory distress	
No			
Dyspnea?	Yes	See separate algorithm	
No			
Productive cough Hemoptysis AND abnormal auscultation AND **Chest pain** or **dyspnea**?	Yes	Pneumonia, TB, pulmonary embolism (systemic signs)	ER
AND weight loss, OR hx smoking, OR hx cancer?	Yes	Lung cancer, lung metastases (CA warning signs, hx cancer)	Urgent
No			

COUGH CONTINUED

Accompanying Signs or Symptoms		Potential Condition (and Confirmatory S&S)	Action
Hemoptysis AND normal auscultation?	Yes	Lung cancer, lung metastases (CA warning signs, hx of cancer)	Urgent
		Throat, nasopharynx, bronchial injury (hx trauma)	Urgent (if airway is clear)
No			
Purulent sputum AND abnormal auscultation?	Yes	Pulmonary infection, pneumonia, bronchitis, bronchiectasis (fever usually present)	Urgent or ER
No			
Purulent sputum AND normal auscultation?	Yes	Pulmonary or nasopharangeal infection (tonsillitis, pharyngitis)	Urgent
No			
Clear or mucoid sputum?	Yes	URI, asthma, allergy, coryza (auscultation normal, no fever)	Standard
AND abnormal auscultaton?	Yes	Manage as "purulent sputum with normal auscultation," above	Urgent
No			
Nonproductive cough			
Back or **chest pain**?	Yes	Aortic aneurysm (pulsing SC joint, syncope, changing vital signs, or hx/morphology of Marfan's syndrome)	ER
No			
Lymphadenitis (cervical)?	Yes	Nasopharyngeal infection	Urgent
AND systemic signs?	Yes	Lung cancer or pulmonary infection (auscultation abnormal)	Urgent
No			
Sore throat, sneezing, rhinorrhea, low fever?	Yes	Coryza or URI (auscultation normal)	Standard
No			
Recurs after exercise only?	Yes	EIB (clear in 20 minutes, postexercise cough)	Standard
No			
Hx of allergy, asthma?	Yes	Asthma, bronchospasm (expiratory wheezing, tight chest; see also **dyspnea**)	Standard
No			
Hx of smoking?	Yes	Smoker's cough (morning cough worse)	Standard

Automatic ER if: ABCs impaired; cyanosis; sudden and severe onset. Urgent or ER if: vital signs stable, fever < 101°F, and no respiratory distress (cyanosis, anxiety); urgent referral is appropriate.

DIARRHEA

Accompanying Signs or Symptoms		Potential condition (and Confirmatory S&S)	Action
Fever?	Yes	See separate algorithm.	
No			
Abdominal pain AND rigidity, OR distention OR ileus	Yes	Bowel obstruction, perforation	ER
No			
Red blood in stool			
AND pus in stool, **abdominal pain?**	Yes	Dysentery (**fever** usually present) or ulcerative colitis (severe dehydration = ER)	Urgent
No			
AND **vomiting**, abdominal cramps beginning 1 to 6 hrs after eating?	Yes	Food poisoning	Urgent
No			
AND perianal/rectal trauma	Yes	Rectal or perianal tissue injury	Urgent
No			
AND hx hemorrhoids?	Yes	Thrombosed hemorrhoid	Standard
No			
Melena (black, tarry stool)?	Yes	Ulcer or other upper GI bleeding (cyclic **abdominal pain** after meals) OR ingestion of cherries, iron, bismuth within previous 24 hrs	Urgent None (if clears)
No			
Acute, nonbloody, loose stool			
AND **vomiting**, pain umbilical, OR McBurney's, OR rebound tenderness, OR positive "jar" sign?	Yes	Appendicitis, peritonitis	ER
No			
AND **vomiting**, myalgia, but no **abdominal pain**, tenderness, rigidity?	Yes	Viral gastroenteritis (should resolve in <48 hrs, usually a fever; maintain hydration)	Standard
No			
AND recurrent **vomiting?**	Yes	Food poisoning (symptoms usually occur within 6 hrs of eating)	Standard
No			
AND hx alcohol or drugs (antibiotics, vitamin C, laxatives) in previous 24 hrs?	Yes	Pharmacologically increased peristalsis (screen for substance abuse; eating disorder if laxatives are abused)	Standard
No			

Diarrhea continued

Accompanying Signs or Symptoms		Potential Condition (and Confirmatory S&S)	Action
Chronic, nonbloody, loose stool			
AND fatty/greasy stool	Yes	Pancreatitis (hx of alcohol abuse or cholelithiasis)	Urgent
No			
AND **abdominal pain**, weight loss, borborygmi (audible peristalsis)	Yes	Inflammatory bowel disease	Urgent
	Yes		
No			
AND abdominal cramps, anxiety, but no weight loss?		Irritable bowel syndrome	Standard
No			
AND abdominal cramps, but no tenderness or rigidity?	Yes	Food allergy (seafood, milk, cereal, MSG), only when ingesting offending food	Standard

Dyspnea

Accompanying Signs or Symptoms		Potential Condition (and Confirmatory S&S)	Action
Chest pain?	Yes	See separate algorithm.	
No			
Fever?	Yes	See separate algorithm.	
No			
Inspiratory stridor	Yes	Airway obstruction (unable to speak) OR exercise-induced anaphylaxis (croupy cough, signs of shock)	ER
No			
Onset after chest trauma?	Yes		ER
Asymmetrical chest movement?	Yes	Flail chest injury	
Deviated trachea?	Yes	Pneumothorax, atelectasis (auscultation and percussion abnormal)	
Subcutaneous air (crepitus)	Yes	Pseudomediastinum, pneumothorax	
Positive compression test?	Yes	Rib fracture	
No			
Cyanosis, tachypnea, accessory muscle use, difficult speech	Yes	Respiratory distress syndrome (auscultation abnormal)	ER
No			
Productive **cough** AND auscultation abnormal AND			

DYSPNEA CONTINUED

Accompanying Signs or Symptoms		Potential Condition (and Confirmatory S&S)	Action
Fever?	Yes	Pulmonary infection	ER
Chest pain?	Yes	Endocarditis, heart failure	ER
Neither?	Yes	Potential heart failure (hx cardiac?)	ER
No			
Expiratory wheezing?	Yes	Bronchospasm: asthma (hx asthma, panting speech, can't hold breath)	Urgent
		Bronchospasm: exercise-induced (hx postexercise cough, condition resolves 20 to 30 min)	Urgent
No			
Hyperventilation, able to speak	Yes	Anxiety attack (normal auscultation; resolves with psychoemotional calming)	Standard

DYSURIA OR HEMATURIA

Accompanying Signs or Symptoms		Potential Condition (and Confirmatory S&S)	Action
Fever?	Yes	See separate algorithm.	
No			
Recent flank, back, or abdominal trauma?	Yes	Renal or bladder injury (progresses to shock)	ER
No			
Hx hemophilia OR sickle-cell disease OR other blood disease?	Yes	Clotting disorder	ER
No			
Age > 55 AND positive urine dipstick?	Yes	Renal or urinary tract disease	Urgent
No			
Flank, back, or **abdominal pain**			
<u>Age < 15</u> AND **fever**, hypertension?	Yes	Nephroblastoma	Urgent
No			
<u>Age > 15</u> And constant, excruciating, "colic" type pain?	Yes	Kidney stone (disabling pain, **vomiting**)	ER
No			
Mild to moderate?	Yes	UTI, STD, renal infection (**fever**)	Urgent
No			
Cloudy or purulent urine?	Yes	UTI, STD	Urgent
No			

DYSURIA OR HEMATURIA CONTINUED

Accompanying Signs or Symptoms		Potential Condition (and Confirmatory S&S)	Action
Nocturia, male, age > 40?	Yes	Prostatitis, prostate disease	Urgent
No			
Genital or perianal trauma?	Yes	Urethral injury, bladder injury	ER/Urgent
No			
Prolonged, strenuous exercise, such as long-distance running?	Yes	Bladder or renal microtrauma or ischemic damage (occurs only after exercise)	Standard
No			
Medications (NSAIDs, birth control pills, anticoagulant therapy)?	Yes	Renal side effects	Urgent

FEVER

Accompanying Signs or Symptoms		Potential Condition (and Confirmatory S&S)	Action
Fever over 104°F	Yes	Heat stroke, heat exhaustion (altered consciousness, collapse; over 106°F immediately life-threatening)	ER
No			
High-grade (102°F) AND any of the signs or symptoms listed below			ER

(Note: Most high-grade fevers cause malaise, pallor, tachycardia, hyperpnea, weakness, and loss of appetite in addition to other signs and symptoms)

Accompanying Signs or Symptoms		Potential Condition (and Confirmatory S&S)	Action
Syncope, altered consciousness	Yes	Endocarditis, myocardial infarction, sepsis/septemia, neurological infection	
Severe headache, rigid neck	Yes	Meningitis (positive Kernig or Brudzinski tests)	
Abdominal pain, rigidity	Yes	Peritonitis	
Vomiting or **diarrhea**	Yes	Gastroenteritis, GI infection, food poisoning	
Cough with purulence OR abnormal auscultation	Yes	Pneumonia or other pulmonary infection	
Chest pain And **dyspnea**, cyanosis, or syncope	Yes	Cardiac event or infection	
Joint pain and loss of motion	Yes	Septic arthrosis, metabolic arthrosis, leukemia	
Dysuria, increased urgency	Yes	Urinary infection, renal infections	

Fever Continued

Accompanying Signs or Symptoms		Potential Condition (and Confirmatory S&S)	Action
Unusual bleeding or bruising, or nontender lymphadenitis	Yes	Leukemia, lymphoma	
No			
High-grade (102°F) without any of the signs or symptoms above	Yes	Infection (check temperature every 2 to 4 hrs; if sustained 102°F=ER)	Urgent
No			
Low-grade (99°F to 101.9°F) AND sustained > 48 hrs duration	Yes	A number of conditions, including anemia, endocrine crisis, immune compromise, cancer (assess for other signs)	Urgent
No			
Low-grade AND < 48 hrs duration AND dysuria, increased urgency	Yes	Urinary tract infection	Urgent
No			
Low-grade AND < 48 hrs duration AND severe postoperative joint pain, erythema, sudden loss in motion	Yes	Postoperative infection	Urgent (contact surgeon's office)
No			
Low-grade AND < 48 hrs, AND nonproductive cough, rhinorrhea, normal auscultation	Yes	Upper respiratory infection, coryza (48 hrs duration)	Standard
No			
Any recurrent fever (consecutive days or nights, cyclic)	Yes	Malignancy, other chronic conditions	Urgent

LYMPHADENITIS

Accompanying Signs or Symptoms		Potential Condition (and Confirmatory S&S)	Action
Fever?	Yes	See separate algorithm.	
No			
Age < 20 (any location)?	Yes	Infection	Urgent
No			
Location			
Cervical, unilateral?	Yes	Infection of head, eye, ear, nose, mouth, etc (local S&S to confirm)	Urgent
No			
Cervical, bilateral, AND tender to palpation?	Yes	Mononucleosis	Urgent
No			
AND not tender to palpation?	Yes	Hodgkin's lymphoma, metastases	Urgent
No			
Axillary or inguinal?	Yes	Infection distal to nodes (arms or legs)	Urgent
No			
General lymphadenitis AND fatigue, pallor, arthralgia?	Yes	Rheumatoid arthritis, rheumatic disease	Standard
No			
AND unusual bleeding?	Yes	Leukemia	ER/Urgent
No			
None of the above	Yes	Infection	Standard

VOMITING AND NAUSEA

Accompanying Signs or Symptoms		Potential Condition (and Confirmatory S&S)	Action
Fever?	Yes	See separate algorithm.	
No			
Chest pain?	Yes	See separate algorithm.	
No			
Recent head trauma?	Yes	Rising intracranial pressure (rising BP, decreased HR, usually projectile vomiting without nausea)	ER
No			
Hematemesis (bright red vomiting)?	Yes	Peptic ulcer, gastritis, esophageal varices (varicose veins)	ER
No			
Substantial **abdominal pain** AND rigidity, distention, progressively worse?	Yes	Peritonitis	ER

VOMITING AND NAUSEA CONTINUED

Accompanying Signs or Symptoms		Potential Condition (and Confirmatory S&S)	Action
No AND fecal odor in vomitus, absent bowel sounds?	Yes	Bowel obstruction	ER
No ANDupper abdomenpain and right shoulder pain?	Yes	Cholecystitis, cholelithiasis	ER
No Back or flank pain AND acute hematuria?	Yes	Kidney stone	ER
No AND chronic nocturia, pallor?	Yes	Renal disorder	ER
No Headache AND rigid neck, rising **fever**?	Yes	Meningitis (rapid collapse)	ER
No AND photophobia, phonophobia, no systemic signs?	Yes	Migraine headache (hx recurrence)	Standard
No Cyclic pain with diarrhea OR loss of appetite OR borborygmi?	Yes	Food poisoning (hx of eating in restaurant, undercooked food, etc) or gastroenteritis (monitor hydration status)	Urgent
No Female, amenorrhea, weight gain, polyuria?	Yes	Pregnancy (recurrent vomiting in morning; ER if signs of shock)	Standard
No After use of alcohol, aspirin, caffeine, drugs?	Yes	Gastritis, peptic ulcer, drug toxicity (urgent or ER if suspected drug overdose; counseling if illicit drugs or alcohol abuse)	Standard
No Low body weight, obsession with weight or calories, Russell's sign on hands/knuckles, self-induced vomiting	Yes	Disordered eating/eating disorder (body image disturbance, inadequate food intake; secretive; mood or personality disturbances, excessive exercise, compulsiveness about eating habits)	Urgent

ABBREVIATIONS FOR ALGORITHMS

BP = blood pressure
CA = cancer
HA = headache
DVT = deep vein thrombosis
EIB = exercise-induced bronchospasm
GI = gastrointestinal
hx = history of
LLQ = left lower (abdominal) quadrant
LUQ = left upper (abdominal) quadrant
RLQ = right lower (abdominal) quadrant
r/o = rule out (ie, exclude from possibility)
RUQ = right upper (abdominal) quadrant
S & S = signs and symptoms
STD = sexually transmitted disease
TB = tuberculosis
URI = upper respiratory infection
UTI = urinary tract infection

Lab Activities

LAB ACTIVITY 1: TESTING DEEP TENDON REFLEXES

Note: When testing the deep tendon reflexes, the athletic trainer documents absence or presence of the reflex response and symmetry of the reflex response in comparison to the opposite limb. Reflex testing is part of the neurovascular examination of a limb, which often includes sensory testing, muscle testing (myotomal), and inspection for vascular signs (pallor and pulselessness).

Lower Extremity (Achilles' and Patellar)

- The subject sits with the legs hanging relaxed from the edge of a table.
- Palpate to locate the inferior pole of the patella and the patellar tendon. Using the wide side of the reflex hammer's head, strike the patellar tendon just below its origin from the patella.
- Normally, the foot and lower leg should move slightly forward (kick). Test the opposite leg for comparison.
- Next, palpate the Achilles' tendon in the posterior ankle. Lift and maintain the subject's ankle in a neutral or slightly dorsiflexed position. Using the wide side of the reflex hammer's head, strike the patellar tendon just above the insertion of the tendon into the calcaneus.
- Normally, the foot plantarflexes slightly, which can be palpated by the examiner.
- If the patellar or Achilles' reflexes are very small or absent bilaterally, have the person clench his or her fists tightly or isometrically pull one hand against the other and repeat the test. These maneuvers increase the reflex response.

Upper Extremity (Biceps, Brachioradialis, Triceps)

- The subject sits with both arms relaxed.
- Support the subject's unaffected arm, flexed to 90 degrees, by holding the elbow with one hand and lying the subject's supinated forearm on top of your own. Place the thumb of the hand holding the elbow firmly on the biceps tendon near its insertion on the radius. Using the pointed side of the reflex hammer's head, strike your thumb sharply.
- Normally, the subject's biceps contracts slightly, which can be both observed and palpated.
- Next, in the same support position, rotate the subject's forearm to a neutral position (halfway between supination and pronation). Using the wide side of the reflex hammer's head, strike the brachioradialis tendon near its insertion on the distal lateral radius.
- Normally, the brachioradialis muscle twitches, which is most observable in the muscle belly near the elbow.
- Last, passively support the subject's relaxed arm in slight extension of the shoulder (about 30 degrees). Strike the triceps tendon just proximal to its insertion at the olecranon.
- Normally, the triceps twitches slightly.

Babinski's Test

- The subject is long-sitting with the feet relaxed.
- Stroke the lateral plantar surface of the foot, beginning at the heel and ending by moving lateral to medial across the metatarsal heads.
- The normal response is flexion (plantarflexion) of all toes.
- If the great toe extends (dorsiflexion) and the other toes "fan out" (abduct), the Babinski's test is positive, indicating serious neurological compromise.

LAB ACTIVITY 2: CARDIAC AUSCULTATION

Note: The role of the athletic trainer in performing cardiac auscultation is to identify potential abnormal heart sounds, not to attempt to diagnose cardiac pathology. Thus, distinguishing normal from abnormal heart sounds is important. By auscultating many subjects who have normal heart sounds, abnormal heart sounds will be easier to identify.

- Subject in supine, males without shirt, females wearing sports bra.
- See cardiac auscultation sites shown in Figure L-1.
- Instruct the person to breathe as normally as possible.
- At each location, listen for abnormal heart sounds during several contraction cycles.
- Mitral valve (M): Palpate the apex of the heart, between ribs five and six (fifth intercostal space) about 1 or 2 inches left of the inferior sternum. Auscultate the apex with the diaphragm of the stethoscope.
- After listening to several heart cycles at the apex, move the stethoscope sequentially to: tricuspid valve (T) at inferior right sternal border at fifth intercostal space; aortic valve (A) at superior right sternal border at second intercostal space; and pulmonary valve (P) at superior left sternal border at second intercostal space.
- If no abnormal sounds are heard in supine, have the person lie on his or her left side and again auscultate the apex of the heart, first with the diaphragm and then the bell (the bell is better at detecting high-pitched sounds). Rushing, hissing, or an "extra" sound suggests mitral valve murmur.
- If left sidelying auscultation is normal, have the person sit, lean forward, exhale completely, and hold his or her breath. Auscultate the apex, again with the diaphragm and then the bell. Rushing, hissing, or an "extra" sound suggests aortic murmur. A "rubbing" sound suggests endocardial/pericardial inflammation.
- Last, have the person sit, hold his or her breath, and bear down as if he or she were going to empty his or her bowels (Valsalva's maneuver) as the apex is auscultated. A "clicking" sound suggests potential mitral valve prolapse (see Figure L-1).

Figure L-1. Auscultation sites for the heart and heart valves.

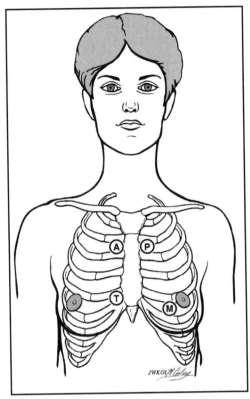

LAB ACTIVITY 3: BLOOD PRESSURE

Note: Much like cardiac auscultation, regular practice greatly improves the ability to assess blood pressure properly (sphygmomanometry).

- The patient and examiner both sit in a quiet area.
- The patient exposes his or her elbow and upper arm.
- Place the cuff around the upper arm such that inflation will occlude the brachial artery (most cuffs are marked with an arrow for placement).
- Place the stethoscope bell over the brachial artery in the cubital fossa (Figure L-2).
- Close the pump valve and inflate the cuff to at least 200 mmHg.
- Slowly release cuff pressure by slightly turning the valve.
- Blood passes the cuff when systolic pressure exceeds cuff pressure on the brachial artery, producing the first sound. The corresponding mmHg is the first or top number in the BP report.
- As cuff pressure continues to decline, the auscultated pulse sounds disappear when diastolic pressure exceeds cuff pressure. The mmHg of the last audible sound is the bottom number in the BP report.
- After completely deflating the cuff and waiting a couple minutes, repeat the measure and report the average readings. Differences in either systolic or diastolic BP greater than 5 mmHg indicate several more trials are needed.

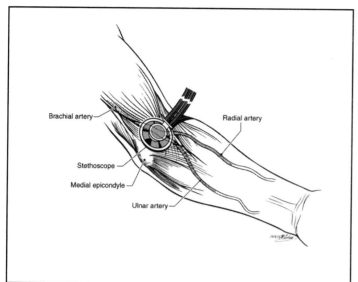

Figure L-2. Stethoscope placement during sphygmomanometry.

Brachial artery

Radial artery

Stethoscope

Medial epicondyle

Ulnar artery

LAB ACTIVITY 4: PULMONARY PERCUSSION

- Male subjects remove shirts, females are in sports bras.
- Begin with subject in supine to inspect the anterior thorax; stand to his or her right side.
- Place the palmar surface of the left distal middle finger on the first percussion/auscultation position (Figure L-3).
- Strike the dorsum of the left finger twice rapidly with the right middle finger, producing quick, solid taps. The normal lung sounds hollow. An "echo" (hyperresonance) or "thud" (pulmonary edema) is abnormal. A more dull sound is heard in the region of the heart (left of the sternum).
- Move sequentially as numbered in Figure L-3, bilaterally comparing identical locations.
- Abnormal findings require emergency (hyperresonance) or urgent (dull) medical care.

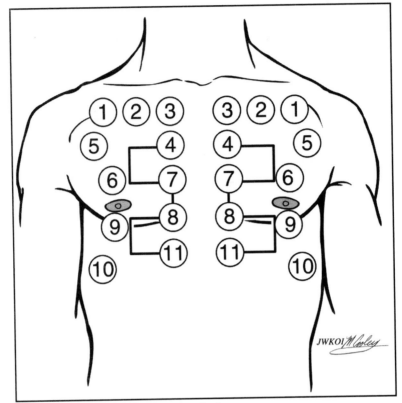

Figure L-3. Percussion points for the lung.

LAB ACTIVITY 5: PULMONARY AUSCULTATION

Note: The role of the athletic trainer in performing pulmonary auscultation is to identify potential abnormal breath sounds, not to attempt to diagnose pulmonary pathology. Thus, distinguishing normal from abnormal breath sounds is important. By auscultating many subjects who have normal breath sounds, abnormal breath sounds will be easier to identify.

- Subject is seated, males with shirt removed and females in sports bra.
- Place stethoscope's earpieces facing posteriorly in the ears.
- The stethoscope's diaphragm is placed on the subject's upper chest (Figure L-4).
- The subject takes a full, deep breath and lets it out slowly and completely.
- Assess sounds upon both inspiration and expiration.
- Repeat in the same location on the opposite side. Progress as in Figure L-4, first over the anterior thorax, followed by the posterior thorax. Slow the pace if the patient hyperventilates or becomes dizzy.
- Identify the tracheal, bronchial, vesicular, and bronchiovesicular sounds in their respective locations (see Figure 4-6). Outside their normal locations, these sounds are abnormal. Complete absence of breath sounds in any location is a medical emergency (probable pneumothorax).

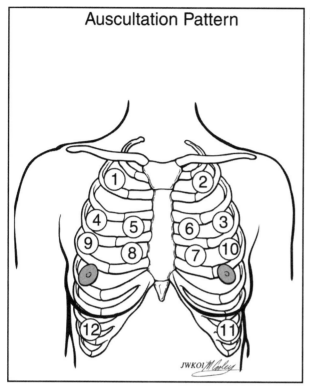

Auscultation Pattern

Figure L-4. Auscultation points for the lung.

- If no abnormalities are noted after auscultating breath sounds across the entire thorax, assess voice sounds in the same locations.
- The subject first speaks and then whispers the long vowels "A" or "E." Spoken sounds are normally muffled but understandable; whispered sounds are normally inaudible. Spoken sounds that are clearly heard or high-pitched, or audible whispered sounds, are abnormal. Hair or movement of costal or vertebral joints can also produce sounds.

LAB ACTIVITY 6: PHYSICAL EXAMINATION OF THE ABDOMEN

- Examine for signs of shock: hypotension, tachycardia, pallor, diaphoresis, altered level of consciousness. If positive, treat for shock and activate EMS (see Chapter Three). If shock is not evident, proceed with physical examination of the abdomen.

Auscultation

- Perform auscultation before disturbing the abdominal contents with palpation.
- The subject is supine with the knees slightly flexed to relax the abdominal muscles.
- Place the diaphragm of the stethoscope flat on the belly.

- Normal bowel sounds are low, irregular gurgling or rumbling noises. Abnormal bowel sounds are like clinking glass or occur as a continuous rumble (hyperactivity).
- "Friction rubs" of peritonitis may be noted over an enlarged spleen or liver.
- Evaluate each region of the abdomen separately.
- Each site should be auscultated for at least 2 or 3 minutes before deciding bowel sounds are absent.
- Absence of bowel sounds in any part of the abdomen suggests a paralyzed section of bowel (ileus), which is a medical emergency.
- Consult Table 5-1 for accompanying signs and symptoms of bowel obstruction.
- Aortic or iliac artery bruits may also be auscultated in the abdomen, usually accompanied by a palpable pulsating mass and signs of cardiovascular pathology (see Chapter Three).

Percussion

- Percussion is performed after auscultation and before palpation. Percussion technique is described in Lab Activity 4.
- Anatomic borders of the liver and spleen may be detectable by percussion. Both organs normally lie mostly behind the lower anterior ribcage (superior to the anterior costal borders).
- Percussion of the liver is performed in the midclavicular (nipple) line from approximately the level of the xiphoid to below the right ribcage.
- The liver is a relatively "solid" organ, approximately 4 to 5 inches in height, and should elicit a dull thud to percussion. See Figure L-5.
- The normal liver's inferior edge is within an inch of the costal border; dullness inferior to this margin suggests hepatomegaly.
- Percussion of the spleen is performed on a line between the midclavicular line and midaxillary line from approximately the level of the xiphoid to below the left ribcage.
- The spleen, relatively "hollow" and much smaller than the liver, should elicit a sound between the "heavy" sound of the liver and the "empty" sound of the bowels, stomach, or lungs.
- When engorged with blood (splenomegaly), a "heavier" sound can be elicited over a much larger area, potentially extending below the umbilicus.
- Most of the abdomen produces a "hollow" sound due to air in the bowels. Ascites (abnormal fluid) sound dull and shift with gravity. Tympanites (excessive air or gas in abdomen) produce a resonant, or hollow, sound.
- If hepatomegaly, splenomegaly, ascites, tympanites, or pain are found upon percussion, stop the physical examination. If the condition was caused by trauma, activate EMS. If nontraumatic, refer the subject for urgent medical examination and testing.
- If these signs are not detected, proceed to palpation.

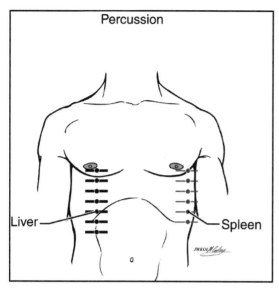

Percussion

Figure L-5. Percussion of the liver and spleen.

Liver — Spleen

Palpation

- Palpation should be performed slowly and gently but firmly enough to penetrate abdominal muscles.

- The palmar surfaces of the distal fingers are used, either a single hand or one hand on top of the other.

- Exert a firm, downward force. Avoid poking suddenly or unevenly, and do not drag the fingers across the skin. Lift and repeat at each location.

- Always palpate the abdomen in the same order to avoid confusion: LUQ (liver and gallbladder), RUQ (spleen, pancreas, and stomach), RLQ (appendix and ascending colon), LLQ (descending colon).

- Pain, rigidity, or rebound tenderness (pain upon sudden release of pressure) are abnormal. If the abdomen is too painful to palpate or too rigid to depress, significant abdominal pathology is very likely.

- Do not force the palpation examination.

- Abdominal organs are normally difficult to discern by palpation, so a palpable mass is likely to be pathological.

- A palpable abdominal pulse that is wider than 2 inches to either side of midline may indicate aortic aneurysm.

LAB ACTIVITY 7: PERCUSSION OF THE KIDNEYS

- The subject is in sitting, standing, or prone.

- Place the palm of the left hand on the left costovertebral angle (where the lower "floating" ribs join the spinal column).

- Sharply strike the dorsum of the left hand with the hypothenar edge of the right fist. This should be just hard enough to produce a dull thud.
- Repeat the test over the right costovertebral angle.
- Abdominal or back pain produced or increased by this test is positive for potential kidney pathology.

LAB ACTIVITY 8: OTOSCOPE EXAMINATION OF THE EAR AND NOSE

Ear

- Seat the subject and conduct external examination of ear (observation, gentle tugging on ear to elicit pain, rub fingers near ear to test hearing).
- The subject tilts his or her head slightly down and away.
- Grasp the superior-posterior edge of the ear and pull gently up and back, steadying both hands on the subject's head.
- Insert the otoscope's disposable speculum (the largest that will fit in the ear; it should sit comfortably in the external ear canal) slowly and straight into the ear canal, monitoring the insertion by watching through the otoscope's viewer.
- Slightly move the otoscope up, down, left, and right to view as much of the tympanic membrane (eardrum) as possible.
- Normally, the ear canal is pale or slightly pink and the tympanic membrane is smooth and translucent. Abnormal findings include swelling, erythema of the canal or eardrum, visible fluid or bubbles behind the tympanic membrane, bleeding (which suggests ruptured tympanic membrane), or a darkened, torn, or abnormally shaped tympanic membrane (usually accompanied by hearing loss).

Nose

- Seat the subject and conduct external examination of the nose (observation, palpation of nasal and facial bones).
- The subject tilts the head slightly back.
- Using the largest disposable otoscope speculum available, gently insert it into the nostril, avoiding contact with the septum (central membrane). Monitor insertion by watching through the viewer.
- Normally, the upper nasal passage is somewhat red. Gentle folds of tissue, called turbinates, should be visible. A thin layer of clear mucous and small hairs should be present. Abnormal findings include fresh or dried blood, purulent mucus, edema of the nasal passage, ulcers, polyps (abnormal bumps), or damage to the septum.

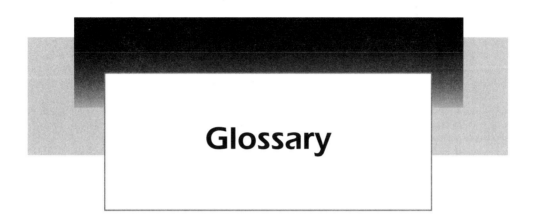

Glossary

This glossary is not a substitute for a good medical dictionary. It is provided merely to facilitate understanding of the material presented in the text.

Phonetic pronunciation of medical terms is in [brackets]. Dashes (-) indicate separation of syllables. CAPS indicate the syllable(s) that is stressed in speech (common medical terms do not include phonetics). For unfamiliar terms, practice pronunciation by reading the phonetic syllables slowly, then repeating them more rapidly until they sound like a single word.

allergy localized, cell-mediated immune reaction to a toxin (ie, an antigen).

alopecia [al-oh-PEE-she-ah] lack of hair in a body region that normally has hair.

amenorrhea [a-MEN-o-REE-uh] lack of menstruation for 3 consecutive months, or less than three menstrual cycles per year; primary amenorrhea occurs when menarche (initiation of menstruation) has not occurred by the age of 16 years.

anaphylaxis [ann-uh-fuh-LACK-sis] generalized inflammatory response, including vascular, pulmonary, and dermatologic systems.

anasarca [ann-uh-SAR-kah] generalized edema; fluid in the interstitial spaces.

anemia [a-NEE-mee-uh] a condition defined as a very low number of circulating red blood cells relative to a person's gender and age group.

angina [ann-JIY-nuh] distinctive type of chest pain that radiates to the arm, neck, jaw, or back, usually lasting 2 to 10 minutes.

anorexia [ann-oh-RECK-see-uh] loss of appetite; occurs with a number of physical, medical, or psychological conditions.

anoxia [ann-OCK-see-uh] lack of oxygen.

antigen [an-tih-jin] a foreign substance that initiates an immune response upon contact with tissue.

anuria [ann-oo-REE-uh] absence of urination.

anxiety a state of intense worry.

arachnodactyly [uh-rack-no-DACK-tee-lee] long, thin fingers ("spider-like").

arrythmia [ah-RITH-mee-uh] interruption of the heart's electrical system, causing an irregular heart beat.

arteriosclerosis [ar-TEER-ee-oh-skleh-ROH-sis] hardening of the arteries.

arthralgia [ar-THRAL-juh] joint pain.

ascites [ah-see-TEEZ] abnormal accumulation of fluid in the peritoneal space of the abdomen.

ataxia [uh-TACK-see-uh] inability to control voluntary movements.

atelectasis [at-uh-LECK-ta-sis] complete removal of air from a segment of lung tissue.

atherosclerosis [ATH-er-oh-skleh-ROW-sis] lipid deposits on the interior of the blood vessels causing a narrowing of the vascular lumen.

atopy [AT-oh-pee] allergy-producing symptoms upon exposure to an offending antigen.

atrophy [AT-ruh-fee] decrease in cell tissue size caused by a decrease in metabolic supply or metabolic demand.

auscultation [AWS-kuhl-TAY-shun] use of a stethoscope to listen for sounds originating in, or conducted by, the body.

benign [beh-NINE] mild, relatively harmless (opposite of malignant).

blood-brain barrier impermeable membrane of the brain's vascular system that prevents diffusion of certain compounds into the central nervous system.

borborgymi [bohr-BOHR-gah-mee] audible grumbling of the bowels.

bradycardia [brayd-ee-KAR-dee-uh] heart rate relatively slower than normal, usually less than 60 beats per minute; may occur at rest in healthy athletes as a result of training.

bronchiolectasis [brong-kee-o-LEK-tah-sis] abnormal increase in the diameter of the bronchus and consolidation of smaller bronchi due to the disease process.

bronchophony [brong-KOFF-ah-nee] abnormal auscultation; spoken sounds are clearly heard.

bruit [BREW-ay] abnormal sound upon auscultation, particularly one detected over an artery.

cancer proliferation of undifferentiated cells replacing normal cells at a high rate of division; malignant dysplasia.

carcinogen [KAR-sih-noh-jihn] a substance known to cause cancer in human tissue.

cardiac hypertrophy [hi-PER-tra-fee] abnormal enlargement of all or part of the heart structures.

cardiac output the product of stroke volume and heart rate; the amount of blood ejected by the heart in 1 minute.

catabolism [kah-TAB-ah-liz-um] metabolic breakdown of cells and tissues.

cerumen [sih-ROO-min] waxy substance secreted in the external auditory canal.

chief complaints symptoms causing an injured or ill person to seek medical attention.

cilia [SIHL-ee-uh] small hair-like projections, particularly on cells lining the airway.

claudication [KLAW-dih-KAY-shun] impairment of gait (ie, limping) caused by vascular pathology.

clinical decision-making determining the best medical course of action for a patient based on history, signs, and symptoms.

clinical diagnosis the identification of an injury, illness, or disease based primarily on medical history and physical examination, without laboratory tests or imaging studies.

clinical pathology the medical practice of pathology as it pertains to the care of patients.

clonus [KLOH-nus] abnormal reflex elicited by sudden flexion or extension of a distal joint and demonstrated by rapid oscillations.

coexisting condition a medical condition in addition to the one for which the patient is seeking care (see also comorbidity).

colic [KAH-lick] a very sudden attack of severe abdominal pain, characteristic of spasm of an obstructed abdominal organ (adj., colicky).

coma [KOH-ma] a complete, profound, and persistent loss of consciousness from which a person cannot be aroused (compare with lethargy).

communicable [kah-MEW-ni-kah-bal] a disease that can be passed directly from person to person, person to animal, or animal to person.

comorbidity [kah-mor-BID-ih-tee] the simultaneous existence of two or more pathological conditions in one person (see also coexisting condition).

concussion collision of the brain with the cranium, causing temporary interruption of neural function.

contagious [kon-TAY-jus] a disease that can be directly passed from person to person.

contrecoup [KON-tra-KEW] concussion occurring opposite the side of impact to the head.

cor pulmonale [KOR PUL-moh-NAHL-ee] right ventricular hypertrophy resulting from increased pulmonary tension, eventually leading to congestive heart failure.

coryza [koh-RIH-zah] "common cold" or rhinitis; accompanied by nasal drainage, sore throat, sneezing, and sinusitis.

cough forceful, often involuntary, expiratory effort, usually to clear the airway of sputum or other substances or objects.

croup [kroop] high, resonant cough, often described as "barking," accompanied by loud, labored breathing, usually associated with laryngeal obstruction.

cyanosis [sigh-ah-NO-sis] bluish tint to the skin; characterized as either peripheral (in the extremities) or central (present throughout the body, particulary the lips, tongue, and face); caused by insufficient oxygenation of the blood.

dermatome [DER-muh-tome] area of cutaneous sensation supplied by one spinal nerve root.

diagnosis definitive identification of an injury, illness, or disease.

diagnostic reasoning identifying and interpreting signs and symptoms to obtain a diagnosis.

diaphoresis [DIE-uh-four-EE-sis] profuse sweating not caused by physical exertion.

diarrhea [die-uh-REE-uh] more than three bowel movements per day, or an unexpected increase in frequency of bowel movements.

diastole [die-AS-toe-lee] passive filling phase of the cardiac contraction cycle.

differential diagnosis determination of which specific disease a patient has.

differentiation sorting and interpretation of signs, symptoms, and other information.

diplopia [die-PLOH-pee-uh] blurred or "double" vision.

disease disruption of homeostasis caused by cellular damage or abnormal organ function.

dysarthria [dis-AR-three-uh] difficulty speaking.

dyspareunia [dis-pa-RUE-nee-uh] painful intercourse.

dysphagia [dis-FA-jee-uh] difficulty swallowing.

dysplasia [dis-PLAY-zee-uh] change of normal cells to several abnormal types with increased rate of division.

dyspnea [DISP-nee-uh] difficulty breathing or "shortness of breath."

dysuria [dis-YOU-ree-uh] painful or difficult urination.

ecchymosis [EK-ih-MO-sis] very dark red, blue, or black discoloration of the skin, caused by blood cells in the interstitial space; a "bruise."

edema [ah-DEE-muh] collection of fluid in a body cavity or interstitial space.

egophony [eh-GOF-oh-nee] abnormal auscultation; spoken sound is transmitted in a high pitch.

embolism [EM-bo-liz-im] sudden obstruction of a blood vessel by an embolus.

embolus [EM-bo-lis] an abnormal particle or object (air bubble, blood clot) freely floating in the blood.

emesis [EM-eh-sus] vomiting.

endocardium [EN-doe-KAHR-dee-um] connective tissue sac that surrounds and invests the structures of the heart.

endothelium [EN-doe-THEE-lee-um] cells lining the cardiovascular system, including the heart, arteries, and veins (see also epithelium).

epistaxis [ep-uh-STACK-sis] nose bleed.

epithelium [EP-ih-THEE-lee-um] cells lining the interior cavities and exterior surfaces of the body (see also endothelium).

erythema [er-ih-THEE-mah] reddening of the skin, usually a result of inflammation.

etiology [eh-tee-AHL-oh-jee] the study of pathogenesis, including theories of illness and disease.

euphoria [yew-FOH-ree-uh] a sensation of pleasant relaxation or well-being.

exacerbated [EKS-as-ur-BAY-tihd] increase in intensity or severity of a disease.

fatigue state of metabolic imbalance that occurs when energy demands exceed energy supply.

fever systemic increase in body temperature; "low-grade" fever is less than 102°F; "high-grade" fever is equal to or greater than 102°F.

gluconeogenesis [GLUE-koh-nee-oh-JIN-uh-sis] conversion of fat or protein to glucose in the liver.

glucosuria [glue-koh-SUE-ree-uh] presence of glucose in the urine.

goiter [GOY-tur] an abnormally enlarged thyroid gland.

gonads organs of reproduction.

gynecomastia [GUY-nih-coh-MASS-tee-ah] feminization of the female breast, including development of mammary glands.

heart failure inability of the heart to maintain normal cardiac output.

hematemesis [HEE-mih-TIM-ee-sis] bloody vomitus.

hematochezia [HIM-ah-toh-KEE-zee-ah] presence of blood in the feces or during defecation.

hematoma [HEE-mah-TOH-mah] collection of blood outside the vascular system.

hematuria [HEE-muh-TUR-ee-uh] blood in the urine, in either microscopic or grossly visible amounts.

hemoglobinuria [HEE-moh-gloh-bih-NEW-ree-uh] hemoglobin in the urine, producing a reddish tint.

hemoptysis [hih-MOP-tih-sis] coughing or spitting bloody sputum.

hemorrhage [HEM-uh-ridj] sudden loss of blood (either internally or externally) resulting from damage to the vascular system.

hemorrhoids [HEM-ih-roydz] varicose veins in the rectum or on the anus.

hemospermia [HE-mo-SPER-me-uh] blood in the male ejaculate.

hepatomegaly [hih-PAT-uh-MEG-uh-lee] pathologic enlargement of the liver.

hernia [HER-nee-ah] a condition in which an organ or part of an organ protrudes through a defect in the wall of the body cavity that normally contains that organ.

hirsutism [HIR-sue-tiz-um] appearance of coarse hair on the chest and face of females caused by abnormal concentrations of androgens from endocrine disorders or anabolic steroid abuse.

homeostasis [HOH-mee-oh-STAY-sis] a healthy state of biochemical dynamic equilibrium within the body's internal environment.

host an organism harboring an infectious agent.

hydrocele [HI-droh-seel] fluid-filled sac in the scrotum.

hypercapnia [hi-pur-KAP-nee-uh] increased carbon dioxide levels in the blood.

hyperhydrosis [hi-pur-hi-DRO-sis] excessive global or localized sweating (eg, the palms of the hands).

hyperlipidemia [hi-pur-lip-ih-DEEM-ee-ah] excessive fat (lipids) in the bloodstream.

hyperplasia [hi-pur-PLAY-see-ah] increase in the total number of cells in a given tissue.

hyperpnea [hi-PERP-nee-uh] rapid ventilation rate.

hypertension high blood pressure; usually systolic over 140 mmHg or diastolic over 90 mmHg.

hyperthermia central body temperature above 37.2°C (99°F).

hypertrophy [hi-PUR-tro-fee] increase in cell size, causing an associated increase in tissue size, resulting from increased metabolic demand.

hyperventilation increase in ventilatory rate without an increase in ventilatory depth.

hypervolemia [HI-pur-voh-LEE-mee-ah] abnormally high retention of fluid in the bloodstream; eventually produces hypertension.

hypopnea [hi-POP-nee-uh] slow, shallow breathing.

hypotension low blood pressure; usually systolic below 95 mmHg or diastolic below 60 mmHg.

hypothermia central body temperature below 32°C (94°F).

hypoxemia [HI-pock-SEE-mee-ah] reduced oxygen saturation in arterial blood.

hypoxia [hi-POK-see-ah] reduced availability of oxygen to the tissues.

icterus [ICK-tur-us] yellow discoloration of the sclera, skin, and mucous membranes; also called jaundice.

idiopathic [ID-ee-oh-PATH-ick] without a known etiology; occurring spontaneously.

ileus [ILL-ee-us] paralyzed section of bowel, usually a result of obstruction or infarction.

impotence [IM-poh-tense] also called erectile dysfunction; inability to achieve or maintain an erection.

incontinence [in-KON-ti-nens] loss of the ability to control either urination or defecation.

incubation time interval between infection and appearance of symptoms.

insidious [in-SID-ee-us] very gradual and unnoticeable progression of disease.

inspection careful observation of a patient to detect signs of pathology.

interstitial [IN-ter-STISH-al] space between cells containing extracellular fluid.

ischemia [iss-KEE-mee-ah] loss of blood flow to a tissue.

jaundice [JAWN-dis] yellow discoloration of the sclera, skin, and mucous membranes; also called icterus.

lability [lah-BILL-ih-tee] instability, unsteadiness, particularly used to refer to mood.

lethargy [LETH-ar-jee] a profound sleep or extreme fatigue accompanying or following disease state; differentiated from coma in that the person can be aroused.

leukocytes [LEW-koh-siyts] white blood cells (phagocytes, eosinophils, etc).

libido [lih-BEE-doh] normal hormonal and emotional sex drive.

lipolysis [liy-POLE-eye-sis] metabolic breakdown of stored fat in response to energy demand (eg, during exercise).

lymphadenitis [LIM-fad-ih-NIY-tiss] swelling of the lymph nodes.

lymphadenopathy [lim-fad-ih-NOP-ah-thee] enlargement of the lymph nodes; a sign of possible infection.

malaise [mah-LAYZ] general discomfort; "not feeling well."

malignant [mah-LIG-nant] severe and harmful; resistant to treatment; highly invasive and pervasive.

medical history status of the person, past and present, related to the current illness.

melena [mel-EE-nah] black stools with the consistency of tar.

menarche [meh-NAR-kee] first menses.

meninges [meh-NIN-jeez] protective layers of connective tissue surrounding the central nervous system.

menses [MEN-seez] sloughing of endometrial lining, consisting of mucous and blood, from uterus through the vagina.

metabolism [ma-TAB-a-LIZ-im] interrelated biochemical functions and processes of the organ systems.

metaplasia [met-ah-PLAY-zee-ah] replacing of one cell type by another.

metastasis [mih-TAS-tah-sis] migration of malignant cells to organs and systems other than those of origin.

myalgia [my-AL-jah] muscular aching.

myocardial [MY-oh-KAR-dee-al] **infarction** ischemic damage to the myocardium; a "heart attack."

myocardium [MY-oh-KAR-dee-um] muscle tissue which comprises the heart; distinct from striated (skeletal) and smooth (organ) muscle.

myoglobulinuria [MY-oh-GLOHB-ew-lin-EW-ree-ah] myoglobin in the urine, a result of excessive exercise and muscle breakdown.

myotomal [my-oh-TOH-mal] groups of muscles controlled by a single nerve root.

necrosis [nih-KROH-sis] metabolic death in a group of cells.

neoplasm [nee-oh-PLAH-zum] tumor; abnormal cell proliferation.

nociceptor [NO-si-SEP-tor] a receptor for pain caused by injury to body tissues.

nocturia [nock-TEW-ree-ah] unusual urgency to urinate, waking the person from sleep.

occult [oh-KULT] hidden, undetected, or undiagnosed.

oligomenorrhea [AHL-ee-goh-men-oh-REE-ah] three to six menstrual cycles per year, with cycles in excess of 35 days.

oliguria [AHL-ee-GEW-ree-ah] very infrequent urination.

orthopnea [or-thop-NEE-ah] dyspnea (shortness of breath) exacerbated when the trunk is upright (as in sitting or standing).

overdose ingestion of toxic amounts of a chemical compound, usually used to indicate poisoning as a result of drug use or abuse.

ovulation [oh-voo-LAY-shun] release of an ovum from the ovary; part of the menstrual cycle.

pain a sensory and emotionally unpleasant symptom, usually associated with tissue damage.

pallor [PAL-or] general paleness of skin caused by vasoconstriction, fever, or vascular collapse.

palpation [pal-PA-shen] manual touch or manipulation conducted during the physical examination.

palpitation [pal-pih-TAY-shun] uncomfortable sensation of forceful, rapid, or fluttering heartbeats.

paresthesia [pair-es-THEE-zah] abnormal cutaneous sensation, including numbness, tingling, burning, etc.

pathogenesis [PATH-o-JIN-a-sis] the cause of a particular disease or morbid process.

pathology 1. medical science concerned with all aspects of disease. 2. the structural and functional changes that result from disease.

pathophysiology [PATH-o-FIZ-e-OL-ah-jee] the physiology of disease.

pectus carinatum [KAR-nay-tum] abnormal convexity of the sternum and anterior ribs; also called "pigeon-chest."

pectus excavatum [ex-kah-VAH-tum] abnormal concavity of the sternum and anterior ribs; also called "funnel-chest."

percussion striking to cause vibration in the internal structures of the body.

pericardium [PER-ih-KAR-dee-um] a double-walled sac of connective tissue that surrounds the heart and its great vessels; contains the pericardial fluid; attaches the endocardium to the thorax.

peritoneum [PAIR-ee-toh-NEE-um] connective tissue lining the abdomen and abdominal organs.

peritonitis [pair-EE-toh-NIH-tis] inflammation of the peritoneum, usually a result of infection (primary) or trauma (secondary).

phagocyte [FAHG-oh-siyt] white blood cells that destroy and ingest foreign microorganisms and cell debris.

phagocytosis [FAHG-oh-siy-TOH-sis] process of ingesting foreign microorganisms and cell debris.

piles hemorrhoids; varicose veins in the rectum or on the anus.

pleura [PLEWR-ah] the sacs of connective tissue lining the thorax and the surface of the lungs; they contain fluid to reduce the friction between the inspiring lung and the chest wall.

pleurisy [PLEWR-ih-see] pain resulting from inflammation of the pleura; sharp and localized, occurring over the affected region.

pleuritic [PLEW-rit-ik] pain similar to that caused by pleurisy; pain over the affected pleural region that worsens during respiration.

pneumoconiosis [NEW-moh-KO-nee-OH-sis] lung disease resulting from chronic inhalation of insoluble or semisoluble particles causing fibrous scarring within the lung.

pneumothorax [NEW-mo-THOR-aks] air or gas in the pleural space (between the visceral and parietal pleura of the lung) causing widespread collapse of the aveoli.

polydipsia [pahl-ee-DIP-see-ah] excessive thirst, usually a result of dehydration or loss of blood volume.

polyphagia [pahl-ee-FAY-jee-ah] excessive intake of food.

polyuria [pahl-ee-EW-ree-ah] excessive frequency or volume of urine.

postprandial [post-PRAN-dee-ahl] relating to the period following a meal.

prandial [PRAN-dee-ahl] relating to the period during a meal.

preparticipation examination physical screening, survey of medical history, and review of organ systems conducted before allowing participation in athletics.

prodromal [pro-DROH-mal] relating to a symptom preceding onset of an illness.

prognosis predicted outcome of injury, illness, or disease.

prostatitis [prahs-tah-TIY-tis] inflammation of the prostate gland.

proteinuria [pro-tay-NEW-ree-ah] presence of protein in the urine.

pruritis [prew-RIY-tis] severe itching.

ptosis [TOH-sis] sagging of the upper eyelids as a result of muscle or nerve dysfunction.

purulent [PYEW-roo-lent] the presence of a thick fluid (also known as pus) containing leukocytes, dead cells, and other tissue debris.

rales [rahlz] also called crackles; abnormal auscultation or a series of distinct pops during inspiration.

rebound tenderness pain elicited upon sudden release of a manually depressed abdomen.

relapse recurrence of an active disease that was previously in remission.

remission absence of detectable or active disease in a person who previously demonstrated the disease; often used to refer to recovery from cancer.

renin [REE-nin] hormone secreted by the kidneys; renin increases vasoconstriction and, thus, raises blood pressure.

respiration exchange of oxygen and carbon dioxide between the circulatory system and the atmosphere; occurs in the aveoli of the lung.

review of systems screening examination of each major organ system; usually conducted by survey or during the medical history.

rhoncus [RON-kus] abnormal auscultation of continuous rumbling during inspiration and expiration.

rigidity "splinting"; protective muscular spasm, particularly of the abdominal wall.

sanguineous [san-GWIN-ee-us] bloody discharge or drainage of body fluid.

seizure sudden electrochemical discharge in the brain causing interruption or alteration of normal cerebral activity.

septicemia [sep-tih-SEE-mih-ah] presence of an infectious organism in the blood.

septum a wall of tissue that divides an organ, such as the heart, into chambers or sections.

serosanguineous [SEE-roh-san-GWIN-ee-us] a combination of watery and bloody discharge or drainage of body fluid.

serous [SEER-us] watery discharge or drainage of body fluids.

shock sudden and severe impairment of the life-sustaining functions of the body; signs include tachycardia, hypotension, diaphoresis, and altered level of consciousness.

sign any indication of pathology observed by the clinician.

smooth muscle muscle tissue of various internal organ systems, such as the gastrointestinal system.

spasm involuntary continuous contraction of skeletal or smooth muscle.

spirometer [spir-AHM-ah-tur] instrument used to measure ventilatory volumes.

splenomegaly [SPLEH-noh-MEG-ah-lee] pathological enlargement of the spleen.

sputum [SPEW-tum] fluid expelled from the mouth during spitting, coughing, or sneezing.

stool feces.

stria [STRY-ah] longitudinal cutaneous discolorations caused by a constant stretch on the skin, such as occurs during pregnancy.

striated muscle muscle tissue which moves the bony skeleton.

stridor [STRY-dur] raspy sound upon inspiration, usually indicative of a partially obstructed airway; usually detectable without auscultation.

stroke volume amount of blood ejected into the aorta during a single ventricular contraction.

symptom any departure from normal function, appearance, or sensation experienced and reported by the patient.

syncope [SIN-koh-pee] complete loss of consciousness and postural tone, caused by a sudden reduction in blood supply to the brain.

systole [SIS-toh-lee] active contraction phase of the cardiac cycle.

tachycardia [tack-ih-KAR-dee-ah] rapid heart rate, usually in excess of 100 beats per minute.

tachypnea [tack-IP-nee-ah] rapid respiration rate; may be in excess of 20 breaths per minute.

thrombosis [throm-BO-sis] formation of a blood clot in a blood vessel.

thrombus [THROM-bas] a clot of blood attached to the wall of a blood vessel.

triage [TREE-ahj] initial examination of a patient to determine the severity of his/her condition.

tumor neoplasm; abnormal cell proliferation.

tympanites [TIM-pah-NEE-teez] abnormal air or gas within the abdomen.

urinalysis [yew-rih-NAL-ee-sis] laboratory analysis of the chemical composition of urine.

urolithiasis [YEW-roh-lih-THI-ay-sis] kidney stone.

urticaria [UR-ti-KAR-ee-uh] hives; lesions of the skin characterized by red, raised regions, usually widespread in reaction to anaphylactic or allergic reaction.

varices [VAR-ih-seez] pathologically dilated veins; "varicose veins."

varicoceles [VAR-ih-koh-seel] varicose veins in the scrotum.

varicose [VAR-ih-kohs] permanently dilated veins.

vector an organism, usually an insect or animal, that passes an infectious organism from one host to another without being affected.

ventilation physical movement of air into and out of the lungs.

verrucae [veh-ROO-sah] warts; tumorous skin lesion caused by papillomavirus.

virulent [VEER-yu-lint] the relative severity, progression, noxiousness, or toxicity of a disease.

vital signs heart rate, respiration rate, blood pressure, and body temperature.

wheals [wheelz] hives; inflammed, raised areas of skin, generally in reaction to an immune response.

whispered pectoriloquy [peck-toh-RIL-oh-kwee] abnormal ausculation; whispered sound is clearly heard.

withdrawal physical and psychological condition produced by the cessation of chronic use of a physically addicting substance.

Index

BUILD *Your Library*

This book and many others on numerous different topics are available from SLACK Incorporated. For further information or a copy of our latest catalog, contact us at:

Professional Book Division
SLACK Incorporated
6900 Grove Road
Thorofare, NJ 08086 USA
Telephone: 1-856-848-1000
1-800-257-8290
Fax: 1-856-853-5991
E-mail: orders@slackinc.com
www.slackbooks.com

We accept most major credit cards and checks or money orders in US dollars drawn on a US bank. Most orders are shipped within 72 hours.

Contact us for information on recent releases, forthcoming titles, and bestsellers. If you have a comment about this title or see a need for a new book, direct your correspondence to the Editorial Director at the above address.

Thank you for your interest and we hope you found this work beneficial.